Postmodern Nursing and Beyond

Cover painting:

Spiritual Energy System from *Sacred Mirrors* series
by Alex Grey 1981.

For Churchill Livingstone:

Senior Commissioning Editor: Alex Mathieson
Head of Project Management: Ewan Halley
Project Development Manager: Valerie Dearing
Design: Judith Wright
Page Makeup: Kate Walshaw

Postmodern Nursing and Beyond

Jean Watson PhD RN FAAN HNC

Distinguished Professor of Nursing, and Founder, Center for Human Caring,
Endowed Chair in Caring Science, University of Colorado,
Health Sciences Center School of Nursing, Denver, Colorado, USA

Foreword by

Barbara Montgomery Dossey RN MS HNC FAAN
Director, Holistic Nursing Consultants, Sante Fe, New Mexico, USA

Larry Dossey MD
Executive Editor, Alternative Therapies in Health and Medicine, California, USA

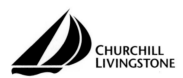
CHURCHILL
LIVINGSTONE

EDINBURGH LONDON NEW YORK PHILADELPHIA SAN FRANCISCO SYDNEY TORONTO 1999

CHURCHILL LIVINGSTONE
An imprint of Harcourt Brace and Company Limited

© Harcourt Brace and Company Limited 1999

 is a registered trademark of Harcourt Brace and Company Limited

The right of Jean Watson to be identified as the author of this work has been asserted by her in accordance with the Copyright, Designs and Patents Act 1988.

First published 1999

ISBN 0 443 05744 3

British Library of Cataloguing in Publication Data
A catalogue record for this book is available from the British Library.

Library of Congress Cataloging in Publication Data
A catalog record for this book is available from the Library of Congress.

Medical knowledge is constantly changing. As new information becomes available, changes in treatment, procedures, equipment and the use of drugs become necessary. The author and the publishers have, as far as it is possible, taken care to ensure that the information given in this text is accurate and up to date. However, readers are strongly advised to confirm that the information, especially with regard to drug usage, complies with latest legislation and standards of practice.

The
publisher's
policy is to use
paper manufactured
from sustainable forests

Printed in China
NPCC/01

Contents

Foreword   vii

Afterword/Dedication   xi

Preface   xiii

Acknowledgements   xvii

Prologue: rewriting self—postmodern meanings   xix

SECTION 1 Transpersonal nursing as ontological *archetype*   1

1 The starting point   3

2 Moving from text to margin   17

3 In search of the sacred feminine: voices from the margins   23

4 Deconstructing modern nursing   33

5 Seeing through Venus's mirror   49

6 Deconstructing modern metaphors   57

7 Reconstructing nursing   75

SECTION 2 Transpersonal nursing as ontological *artist*   91

8 Beyond postmodern nursing—into the next millenium   93

9 Transpersonal caring–healing   105

10 The postmodern/transpersonal body   131

11 The body as a sacred mirror   159

12 Exercises for experiencing the transpersonal body   171

13 Professional ontological competencies for transpersonal practice   177

14 Reconsidering Nightingale: professional ontological competencies as advanced caring–healing arts   201

15 An interlude: the Zen of bedmaking   237

SECTION 3 Transpersonal nursing as ontological *architect* 241

16 Caring–healing architecture within the postmodern/transpersonal 243
paradigm

17 Unconcluding postmodern Nightingale 261

18 Relighting the lamp 269

References 277

Glossary of definitions 285

Index 293

A colour plate section can be found between pages 170–171

Foreword

Something unforeseen and magnificent is happening. Health care, having in our time entered its dark night of the soul, shows signs of emerging, transformed.

Earlier this century, we believed that all the major illnesses and chronic afflictions would yield to the progressive insights of science. In order to usher in the medical utopia, we believed we had only to unravel the physical mechanisms of the body and to focus on physical interventions such as drugs and surgical procedures. Today, however, in spite of the majestic accomplishments of modern medicine, there is a gnawing realization that something has been left out—something vital, something that concerns not the physical function of our bodies but our very being.

'Being' is not a concept discussed in many nursing or medical schools. Neither is 'ontology', that branch of philosophy that deals with the nature of being, reality and ultimates. 'Being' may sound too esoteric to have a place in health care but it is exceedingly practical. In fact, our decisions about how we choose to be constitute a matter of life and death. Consider, for example, that more individuals have fatal heart attacks on Monday morning, between 8 a.m and 9 a.m., than at any other time of the week (the so-called 'Black Monday' syndrome), and that job dissatisfaction has been found to be a potent predictor of first heart attacks. How we choose to *be* in the world—our occupation, our relationships, our priorities and choices—are life-and-death factors, and unless nursing and medicine entertain these 'being' aspects of our lives, they will be incomplete.

This means that it is not enough to focus only on the physical causes of heart disease, such as the major risk factors of smoking, cholesterol, diabetes and high blood pressure; the way we choose to *be* must be considered a risk factor as well.

Jean Watson's book is concerned about these truths. She has discovered —or rediscovered—a central fact about healing that we have forgotten: health care, to be complete, must focus on more than *doing*—it must also address matters of *being*.

Watson's ontological, being-based vision is therefore not 'just philosophy' but is embedded in the everyday. It is also grounded in science. Some may disagree. They may feel that her call for a new model of health care shows ingratitude for a physically based medicine that has saved millions of lives over the past century. But Watson does not discard science, she honors it, builds on it, and extends it. She asks, 'If we have the courage to honor all that science is telling us, what would health care look like? What would it *feel* like to be a patient and a practitioner in a system that honors our very being?'

Watson's vision of transpersonal caring brings back the concepts of 'soul' and 'spirit'. She suggests that there is some quality of human consciousness that cannot be equated with the physical body and which transcends it, and which must be addressed by health care practitioners. For almost the entire span of human history, healers accepted this idea; it is only in the latest heartbeat of history that we have abandoned this concept as unscientific.

In emphasizing the primacy of consciousness, Watson is on firm ground. Leading scientists, mathematicians, and philosophers such as David J Chalmers, C J S Clark, Ervin Laszlo and Nobel prize winner Brian Josephson have begun to consider consciousness as *fundamental* in the universe, perhaps on a par with matter and energy, neither derivable from nor reducible to anything more basic. These are landmark, historic shifts in how we regard the mind, and Watson's views are in accord with them.

About terminology. It is easy to disagree with the language used to express the ontologically based, transpersonal health care interventions.

Critical experiments justifying the literal use of terms such as 'energy fields', 'high-frequency thoughts' and 'negative energy' have, by and large, not been done. As a consequence, these terms may be considered metaphors and images and not reflections of concrete fact. But we should not be too critical. The fact is, the precise nature and origin of consciousness and its relationship to the body and brain are great unknowns. If there is any region within science where images and metaphors should be allowed to float in ambiguity, perhaps this is the area. We need to allow theorists such as Watson immense elbow room—freedom to explore, to try out new ideas, to play with new images and metaphors that may not be accepted when they are first introduced. The history of science can serve as a guide. When Isaac Newton introduced the term 'universal gravity' in the 1600s, his colleagues accused him of surrendering to mysticism. Similarly, when the term 'field' was introduced in physics in the 19th century, it was considered hopelessly murky by some. Precise investigations eventually clarified these new terms, just as they will bring precision to the descriptions of transpersonal caring and healing.

Throughout history, the healing professions have been some of the most dynamic of our social institutions. They have always been in the process of change, as they are currently. Today, then, it is not a question of *whether* the health care professions will change but what the change will be. Jean Watson's vision is a window to these transitions.

How are patients responding? A recent survey of hospitalized patients found that 75% believed their physicians should be concerned with their spiritual welfare, and 50% believed their physicians should pray not just *for* them but *with* them. Currently, three-quarters of family physicians believe spiritual issues are a major factor in their patients' health. Another survey recently found that 40% of working scientists in the USA believe in God. These findings suggest that 'the spiritual' has never really disappeared from healing, and that the chasm between science and spirituality is not as wide as we have thought.

Nurses are at the vanguard of the quickening of the transpersonal currents in healing. This should surprise no one. For centuries, nurses have nurtured and protected the spiritual qualities in health care, often giving their lives in the process. Jean Watson is a standardbearer in this long line of visionaries and heroines, and her message will resonate for a long time to come.

Barbara Montgomery Dossey

Larry Dossey

Afterword/Dedication

Upon completion of this manuscript (June 1997), I suffered a most uncanny accident. As a result, I am now without vision in my left eye and undergoing extensive surgeries and immobilizing treatments. This requires my head being in a downward-flow-facing position 45 minutes of each hour, lying prone on a massage table with my head cradled down. That is what I do. This process will continue for 3 months before I know if my eye can be saved*, if so, then follow-up efforts will begin towards restoring any vision, if possible.

During this time I have had to experience and create my own caring–healing processes for deep, deep healings, even at the cellular level.

Hundreds and thousands of nurses, friends, colleagues and prayer groups around the world have been summoned to pray for my healing and for my family.

As my healing continues and I personally experience my theory of caring, I have many people to thank and I extend my blessings to them.

The first is Douglas, my spiritual and physical partner, best friend, lover, companion, devotee and spouse, who is caring for me as a sacred act, a spiritual practice; he ironically practices my theory of 'postmodern' caring, as I personally benefit from it—from the other side—inside and personal. Also, this work is dedicated to Douglas because he was part of the co-creation of this book. During a Fulbright Research and Lecture

---

*Afternote (January 11, 1998): The eye could not be saved. I am now learning to 'see' anew, myself and surroundings, calling upon my 'third eye' and adjusting to cosmetic prosthesis and a life-changing tragedy–challenge–gift.

Award in Sweden in 1991, he suggested the title of the book—*Postmodern Nursing*—so, intellectually, professionally and at deep personal level I dedicate this work to Doug—my love.**

Further thanks go to my loving family: my daughters Jennifer and Julie and my beautiful grandchildren, who are children for the next millenium—(Jennifer's)—Demitri, 10 years; Alma, 5 years; Theo, 1 year and (Julie's) baby Gabriel, 1 year (at November 1998) and his sister or brother who arrives in April 1999.

They bring me joy and surround me with love, reminding me of the sacred circle of life.

Boulder, Colorado 1997   Jean Watson

**Postscript (August 25, 1998): Doug died in March 1998. He remains a part of my life and this work.

Preface

This work projects nursing and health care into the mid-21st century when there will be radically different requirements for all health practitioners, and entirely different roles and expectations between the public and the health care systems. It presents nursing as a metaphor and paradigm case for women in society, reflecting the imbalance in Western society and Western medicine. It uncovers how modern nursing/medicine has been using only one half, one side, of its brain, so to speak.

Within the dominant, modern, Western mindset, the caring–healing practices of nursing have been on the margins. It is this, the repressed healing capacity of feminine energy, symbolized across time by women in general and nurses in particular—male and female alike—which has been silenced. It is this which is emerging, being reclaimed and rediscovered by nursing and all health professionals as we enter into the next millennium.

Such a reawakening calls forth a model of caring and healing practices which takes medicine, nursing and the public beyond traditional Western medicine, beyond the 'cure at all costs' approach. What is emerging is an entirely different paradigm, based upon a feminine energy rebalancing at the deep archetypal core of our being. Nursing as a metaphor symbolizes this deep, feminine energy, which needs to be expressed at this time.

The essential factor in the event is the archetype, and it is this level that carries the deepest meaning. (Tarnas 1993, p. 6)

These are people who have been pressured into a Yang perspective, who act from that perspective a lot in their daily lives. Yet they can go beyond that to the archetype of healing in the wink of an eye. ... It can always be remembered, reowned.

(Remen 1994)

In addition to the deep archetypal awakenings in humanity, we are being transformed by new and different relationships, languages and experiences. These changes fluctuate between intergalactic space explorations and cyberspace and hyperspace. They move between text and hypertext to hidden text, jumping from 'word processing' to 'thought processing', leaping from text to subtext to intertext; from actual to virtual, no longer aware of differences, no longer dealing with logical, linear thought or data. Such quantum leaps in human experience require that we reconsider our very concept of being.

Ultimately, what is being proposed goes beyond a paradigm shift toward a more fundamental ontological shift. This shift acknowledges another new phenomenon that has emerged in this century, namely the symbiotic relationship between humankind–technology–nature and the larger, expanding universe. This fundamental turn evokes a return to the sacred core of humankind, in relation with the universe, connecting with a sense of the divine and inviting the awe and mystery back into our lives and work. Such thinking holds a sense of reverence and openness for the infinite possibilities contained within both our inner and our outer space. It offers a search for the spiritual aspects of our being and our approaches to health and healing.

This expanded view posits the importance of ontological caring–healing practices (which evoke a different consciousness and intentionality, grounded in the sacred healing arts) now needed to intersect with and realign the dominant, technological treatment capabilities of advanced medical science. The ontological shift affects humankind itself, and the natural human potential and capacity for self-care and self-healing possibilities, yet to be imagined. The ontological shift, combined with a return to the sacred healing arts, is already disrupting, disturbing and displacing conventional medical, nursing and health care practices and practitioners as we know them.

While grounded historically and metaphorically in nursing, and to some extent in Nightingale's original blueprint, the work embodied in this book paradoxically and simultaneously transcends nursing. All current and future health care systems and practitioners are being deconstructed by the proposed ontological shift, inviting and requiring a reconstruction of health care and a revision of all medical and professional health education and practices.

The ontological shift invites practitioners to embark upon the following paths:

- Path of awareness, of awakening to the sacred feminine archetype/cosmology to rebalance the disorder of conventional modern medicine and the modern, cultural mindset.
- Path of cultivation of higher/deeper self and a higher consciousness: transpersonal self.
- Path of honoring the sacred within and without; open to deeper explorations of the mystery of the human body and life-healing processes: postmodern–transpersonal body.
- Path of acknowledging the metaphysical/spiritual level, attending to the non-physical, spiritual dimensions of existence.
- Path of acknowledging quantum concepts and phenomena such as caring–healing energy, intentionality and consciousness, as paths toward expanding human existence and the evolving human consciousness.
- Path of honoring the connectedness of all; unitary consciousness; the eternal 'caring moment'; 'transpersonal caring–healing'.
- Path of honoring the unity of mindbodyspirit; both immanence and transcendence of the human being and becoming.
- Path of reintegrating the caring–healing arts, as an artistry of being, into healing practices: ontological competencies.

- Path of creating healing space: healing architecture.
- Path of a relational ontology, open to new epistemologies of existence.
- Path of moving beyond the modern–postmodern into the open, transpersonal space and the new thinking required for the next millennium.

All health professions are being, and will have to be, redefined for this ontological shift to take place. The new ontologically based practices will not be the exclusive domain of any one health profession, but will affect all. All will have to transform, as they are being symbiotically transformed.

While these ideas may seem marginal, such thinking is already being integrated into the center of mainstream practices. This turn is reflected in the self-directed individual and community, in self-care and self-healing regimes, and in the emerging shifts in science itself (chaos theory, complexity science and quantum physics).

Once the changing worldview and the new models of scientific practice are more fully comprehended, the face of medicine, nursing and health care will never be the same again. In spite of the turmoil of change, the emerging model offers hope and possibilities for a new affirmative order of wholeness which we seek as a people and a civilization.

Sonora, Mexico 1998   Jean Watson

Acknowledgements

First and foremost, my gratitude and most sincere appreciation, respect, awe and thanks to Diane Lenfest of the University of Colorado School of Nursing, for her comprehensive review and application of publication requirements and guidelines. Without Diane's assistance in the final stages of the manuscript, this book might still be in limbo, awaiting final touches for completion.

Diane began her assistance upon my completion of the manuscript and before my accident. Once I was out of commission, so to speak, I relied with trust and full confidence upon Diane's competence and professional standards of excellence. I remain in her debt for her many courtesies. Her gracious, cheerful efforts and hard work were a labor of love, a cherished gift to me and to the work itself.

To Alex Mathieson of Churchill Livingstone I extend my thanks for his encouragement throughout this project. He believed in its importance and engaged in its completion with such personal interest and attention.

Allan Graubard of the National League for Nursing I thank for his early support, critique and feedback, and for his willingness to facilitate international relationships for cooperative marketing and distribution of the work.

My dear friend and colleague, Björn Sjöstrom of Göteborg University in Sweden I thank for his review of earlier versions of the manuscript, and for his helpful suggestions and optimism about the ideas set forth in this work. Our dialogues and discussions both in the USA and Sweden were a source of inspiration to me.

My ever-loyal colleague and friend, Karen Peeters, Executive Director of the Center for Human Caring and angel helper. What can I say? I offer my love and my humble thanks for a million things along the way on a journey we have shared for many years now. We continue to be sojourners walking together into the unknown. Also, to Floyd Curvin, in the Center, a dedicated assistant to and supporter of me personally and of all the Center's goals. To Janet Quinn for her healing energy and power and for holding me in the light.

My thanks to all caring–healing networks of like-minded colleagues and students around the world, who are inspired by nursing's emerging paradigm for a new era. You inspire me and give me hope and confidence that we can make a difference—ideas count, and can transform, as we work together at this turn of the century.

Last, to all my colleagues and loving students at the University of Colorado. My roots and strength come from you. I test out my ideas and benefit from your experiences. The Colorado mountains and the University of Colorado have launched me into the world and around the globe, but I always return to Colorado, where I belong.

To all those whom I cannot name but whom I carry in my heart as you all shape my past and my future. I am blessed.

Prologue: rewriting self —postmodern meanings

....

Journal notes: Friday, February 10, 1995
Sea of Cortez, Mexico

I have been here for 1 week in this sacred space. I write from my heart today. I take in this idyllic jewel on the sea, the winter sun, providing warmth to protect and encompass me; mindbodysoul as one. I have written every day for a week from my head and through the words of others. Today I write for myself; I hear and take in the continuous slapping and rhythmic splashing of the waves on the shoreline outside my door that opens to the sea. The sea eagle soars along the waterline and swoops for fish while the seagull lazily suspends itself on a film of invisible air, leaving it hanging halfway between sea and sky. This view encircles me daily, and nightly the crescent moon hangs above me; today/tonight it will be half full, filling up as I work on this book.

This book has been carried in my mind and has been presented worldwide to different groups of nurses and other professionals. It has evolved over a career of almost 35 years in nursing and it places human caring at the core of the profession. This is something that is yet to be realized or actualized, but is awaiting an awakening as we enter another century and another time in human and nursing's history.

More specifically, this book has been in preparation for the past 5 years. I have not been able to write it until now, and even now I am cautious about my abilities. Do I have the intellectual and conceptual clarity to express the depth of my 'knowing', 'seeing' and wisdom about nursing as I have lived it, shared it, written it, witnessed it and uncovered it as the ground of being, at both a personal and professional level?

Here, I am attempting to rewrite nursing as I rewrite self. There is a saying that you teach what it is you need to learn; so it is probably true of writing. I write to teach myself what it is I need to learn about myself and to express what I need to express. I also wonder what it is I need to learn and express about changing self, and changing nursing, as part of the process of writing.

At a deeper, more intimate level, I am writing and rewriting self as a metaphor for the search for the sacred, the deep-energy, beauty-feminine principle: the raison d'être of life, the living spirit of creation, generativity and the relationship with Mother Nature at this time in the universe, a universe that is preparing for a new era in human history.

My pain is witnessing mainstream, institutional nursing trying so hard and yet being so defeated by institutional oppression, no matter how optimistic, confident and self-enlightened the person or the institution. Nursing struggles both within its inner self and within the outer world; it does not know or is not able to grasp, experience, witness or create its own power with its deep, feminine healing energy of possibilities. It continues to struggle in its attempts, no matter how grand and constructive, to be heard, seen and valued for its strength and its worldview of possibilities. Nursing remains handicapped in its move toward its own authentic model.

On the other hand, my personal and professional joy and privilege come from tapping into the other dimensions of nursing (and myself), and in working worldwide with nurses in these dimensions. It is here that we tap into the collective unconscious of nursing's archetypal soul. It is here, also, that I help myself and others remember what we are here to do, why we are in nursing, and where our life-giving, life-enriching power lies in our work, whether we be educator, researcher, administrator, clinician or consultant.

When individually or collectively nursing enters into its nursing qua nursing ground of being, it brings forth in itself and the profession a new possibility for humankind. Such work, however, is usually a silent backdrop to a much harsher institutional culture, which usurps the healing and regenerative energy of nursing and nurses. Often nurses succumb and are 'bought out' by the mainstream dominant culture, to the neglect of their soul work. When this happens we all suffer as a result. I somehow feel nursing's pain as if it were my own and I must write to deal with this pain. Is it in going through pain that we enter joy?

Together, nursing and I are learning other ways, and that is what this book is all about, at a deep personal level. It also spills over into my hope and message for the next generation of nurses.

Of course, it all depends upon the reader as to how this book will be received and interpreted. Nevertheless, I write it for self, for other nurses and for nursing's future emergence in its own right, not self-righteously, but with poise and natural maturity.

Since 1986, through the establishment of the Center for Human Caring at the University of Colorado, I have been convinced that the caring–healing dimensions of nursing are needed now more than ever, and are emerging as a mature paradigm for nursing science and practice at both the disciplinary and professional level. What I hope to capture here is the nursing qua nursing paradigm that I see as a fuller completion of the model in which nursing has operated all along. This model, however, needs further articulation and explication if it is to be endorsed and accepted both within and without. Otherwise, without seeing this new/old redefined entity called nursing, we are prone to persist with the old debates which make a case for nursing in a model that is already dead. We do not know or see this yet, so we struggle to become part of what no longer is, rather than emerging into our own beauty, like a blossoming flower having come to its time of bloom. As such, it sheds light and beauty and joy to all who see and experience it.

Within the emerging nursing qua nursing paradigm, which I call the transpersonal caring–healing model, nursing is able to draw upon the finest of its art and science. It is able to reclaim and reintegrate at a deeper, higher level the original tenets of Nightingale. It is able to reattend to the unity of mindbodyspirit and to the human/environment oneness of being. It is able to see and experience the power of the caring–healing consciousness, intentionality, ethic, energy, connectedness and wholeness as part of the ground of meaning and being as a person, in caring–healing relationships with self, other, nature and culture itself. These now all cry out for caring–healing, for wholeness, for survival; they call to us to grow and evolve as humans in harmony with and in honor of the universe, rather than dismembering and dishonoring at all levels.

This emerging nursing model is a hopeful solution for healing the nursing profession itself, with its collective wound and long-lost memories of its healing role, but it also becomes a model of possibility for medicine and health care generally. It is about something beyond men and women and medicine and nursing. Nursing is a timeless metaphor for the opportunity within the professional world to reclaim and recapture the sacred feminine of ancient healing practices, while still benefiting and drawing upon the finest of medical and scientific knowledge and technology acquired during this modern era of revolution in medicine and nursing science.

This thinking for nursing goes beyond the modern time, while maintaining the modern tenets that work. In considering postmodern nursing and beyond, the word 'nursing' should really be slashed out to indicate that it is no longer an adequate word for this time of transformation toward caring and healing. It is too embedded with the so-called modern nursing practices, procedures, language and stereotypes which encode and restrict what it is yet to become and must become if it is to mature as a distinct health profession, meeting its unmet expectations to society for the caring–healing so desperately needed for all.

The other meaning of postmodern nursing, with the word 'nursing' slashed through, is to convey that it is past the modern stereotype and industrial, masculine archetypal, patriarchal, medical and institutional thinking. In that modern era, which now has to be transcended, nursing, in its attempt to be helpful and accepted in the dominant culture of its time, took on, participated in and was co-conspirator to practices which no longer accommodate the health and healing needs of people the world over. Perhaps nursing took on these medical orientations unwittingly, but nevertheless we, as the largest collective health profession, have failed to honor our raison d'être and have served the master, masculine archetype script in education and practice in our search for being.

As a profession at a crossroads in its history and in-between time, nursing has yet to actualize itself in a paradigm that goes beyond the deeply masculine archetype of modern medicine. There are, however, some individual exceptions on the horizon. For example, contemporary nursing theory has more clarity as a nursing qua nursing paradigm (which can be seen to be located within a feminine archetype, although that has not been made explicit in nursing theory literature to date).

In nursing research and doctoral programs there are new, non-objectivist models for nursing research, which have great promise for nursing science as a distinct discipline in the university, not simply a subset of medical science or behavioral social science. While nursing has much in common with feminist research, studies of women, educational models in hermeneutics and phenomenological postmodern interpretative inquiry methods, which are now becoming mainstream, nursing is often reluctant to see other disciplines that can provide synergy and support. This is often because nursing is located on biomedical research and medical school campuses or in basic science departments in colleges and universities, keeping it socialized within a dominant science paradigm.

Nevertheless, all this is changing and must change if nursing is going to be anything more than a technical assistant model for an evolving medical science or, if not a technical assistant, then perhaps an ethical or philosophical assistant, but not a distinct health profession which works as a mature partner with other distinct health professions. For some reason, nursing remains under the broader umbrella of medical science and practice. It is time for nursing to raise its own tent and invite others in—a tent that is collapsible and movable from house to house, from community to community, from country to country, from desert to seashore, from mountains to plains.

Groups such as the American Holistic Nursing Association and the International Association of Human Caring have ushered in healing dimensions of nursing long abandoned by 'modern' nursing and 'modern' institutions. Nursing scholars, philosophers and other authors are focusing on caring and nursing ethics and ethos and caring morality, and have contributed to nursing's emergence within its own value/ethical framework. Nursing scholars, feminist writers, faculty doctoral students and other disciplines have been systematically critiquing and deconstructing the fallacy of the dominant traditional and medical science epistemology for human science phenomena, especially with respect to caring and healing practice and human responses, and experiences of health, illness, living, dying, birthing, growing, suffering, learning, evolving, transforming and so on.

Will nursing let medical science be for medical science, even though that is changing as well? For its soul's sake, will nursing own its own science phenomena and stop duplicating medicine at every turn? Or is nursing still, after all, just a subset of medicine, choosing to remain inside its tent, complaining all the while, and withering away its gifts of life and living and healing? Do we, as nurses, drop out and create another way of living? Do we align with other like-minded groups or do we create new models of being for self and others? These are the pressing existential questions of this time in our history. After 100 years can we change, or are we forever condemned to be what we have become?

Even as I despair, I am an eternal optimist and have a vision of what might be and already is beginning to manifest in human consciousness and public health care, and which is totally consistent with the caring–healing model that has always guided nursing, even if unconsciously, often without being recognized or fully developed. In the past 30 years dramatic advances have been made in the consciousness of nursing, nursing science and practice. While we still have some other significant and difficult turns to make towards being and becoming a mature caring–healing profession, we are on our way and making quantum leaps. That is why I write now, to catch this change in action, in the process of its emerging.

One of the next turns for nursing's full emergence is to see the convergence and culmination of the developments over the past 30 to 40 years and to lay out the resulting transformative paradigm of transpersonal caring–healing which comes now from the deep roots of nursing's ancient traditions and beliefs. This paradigm is ready to be actualized but is, ironically, beyond nursing. The caring–healing tradition and emerging model is now converging with other developments in science, progressive medicine and healing professions worldwide. Thus, if clarified and upheld as a hopeful paradigm, it can serve to transform the whole of health care within the postmodern era and move toward the transpersonal for a new century, demanding an evolved consciousness from all its health and healing practitioners.

Just because nursing matures within its model of science and practice, it does not 'own' the paradigm, the insights or knowledge. Just as all health professions within the modern era have practiced under a dominant medical paradigm of consciousness during the 20th century, the nursing caring–healing model can be a model for other practitioners who practice within it (not under it) for the postmodern era and beyond: the next leap in human health history.

The nursing qua nursing model of transpersonal caring–healing more fully accommodates the human–nature–life processes of the mindbody-spirit unity, the art and science which returns a sense of sacred, harmonious, beautiful, ritual, archetypal unity as the ground of our being as healers within a caring–healing profession. We are not mechanics and technicians fixing people and diseases, no matter how well we have been professionalized into acting that way.

A word of caution—the model proposed is not a model for all nurses or all health professionals; some will need to remain in their modern, technical place. There is room for all in this model, but it invites anyone who wishes to engage in the life-giving, life-receiving aspects of its healing work to enter wherever and whenever she or he wishes, or not at all. For those who wish to evolve and emerge as more fully human, caring and compassionate individuals—whatever their field, practice or educational level—the caring–healing model is a model to reach towards. It is qualitatively and consciously different from the modern medical and nursing models. It is also more than just postmodern: it requires a radical transformation of our consciousness, our cosmology and our being in the universe.

> Women have worked into the time spaces of tomorrow to rearrange it in terms of perceived needs of social groups not well served today ... If the phenomenon of the underlife (of women) is a chance detour in the social evolution of the human race—a detour that 'drifted towards the absurd sex role imbalance we note today'—can the evolutionary process be redirected?
>
> (Boulding 1992, pp. 340–341)

Transpersonal nursing as ontological *archetype*

1

The starting point

At this cross-roads ... we cannot stop and wait because we are pushed forward by life ... what are we going freely to decide?

(Teilhard de Chardin 1959, p. 233)

For my people standing, staring, trying to fashion a better way from confusion, from hypocrisy and misunderstanding, trying to fashion a world that will hold all the people, all the faces, all the Adams and Eves and their countless generations.

(Walker 1975, p. 1168)

Crossing from the shore

While Margaret Walker wrote for her people of color, this book is written for nurses and women, for men and medicine. It is written for any who wish to identify with another way of being in relation to self, a way of being which honors the sacred within health and healing. It is for those in the medical health profession, for patients and the public alike, any and all who know the medical system and the culture that informs it and who know and admit that the system is out of order and needs to be rebalanced and realigned.

This book takes the reader on a 'journey' from the modern to the postmodern and beyond. As such it can be interpreted as a 'boat' of sorts, and aims to create a consciousness of how to make the crossing from one century and one millennium to another. Steinbeck (1951), in his Log from the Sea of Cortez, said that out of the essential race-soul[1] came the *boat*. To humankind, a boat, more than any other tool of human use, is a representation of an archetype.

As Steinbeck put it, there is an 'idea', *boat*, that is an emotion, and because the emotion is so strong it is probable that no other tool is made with such honesty. Steinbeck believed that a person builds the best of *self* into a boat, building into it many of the unconscious memories of ancestors and receiving back from it a warping of one's psyche. He observed that there is no counterpoint in nature to a boat, unless it be a dry leaf fallen by accident into a stream.

Steinbeck's archetypal boat symbolizes millenniums of trial and error of the human consciousness. The sight of Steinbeck's boat, riding in the water, clenches an emotion. To make the crossing from one century and one millennium to another, we now have both to *create* and to *be* our own boat.

Used as a 'boat', this book can transport the reader toward and through new ideas and concepts, or the reader can use it to 'fish' for new notions or for a new consciousness. It can be used as a means of going out to sea and seeking connections with the wider, open cosmos—*out there*, in a wider sea of consciousness, open to celestial navigation as the route required to touch the point where the heavens and earth meet at the intersection of time and timelessness.

Using this book as a boat, the reader can also navigate between the shore of the text, which is familiar and solid, and the wider sea of the

---

[1]The intrinsic soul of humanity, of the human race; it also conveys archetypal dimensions of a shared soul of humankind, an enduring form that resides in human consciousness (in this instance 'boat').

margins, tacking back and forth across the water, moving between the text and the margins that float in the water trying to reach the distant shore. Such navigational crossings take us toward the deeper waters of the open sea, full of floating and fluid uncertainties that undulate with the rhythm of another order that is generally unknown and unfamiliar.

While unfamiliar, the far shore and open sea nevertheless beckon us to attempt the crossing, especially at this point in human history.

In Teilhard de Chardin's writings, he too uses sea metaphors:

> *What we are up against is the heavy swell of an unknown sea which we are just entering from behind the cape that protected us. What is troubling us intellectually, politically, and even spiritually is something quite simple ... 'We have only just cast off the last moorings which held us to the Neolithic age' ... We are, at this very moment, passing through a change of age. Beneath a change of age lies a change of thought. Where are we to look for it, where are we to situate this renovating and subtle alteration which, without appreciably changing our bodies, has made new creatures of us? In one place and one only—in a new intuition involving a total change in the physiognomy of the universe in which we move—in other words, in an awakening.* (Teilhard de Chardin 1959, pp. 214–215).

So like a boat, sometimes in tranquil and sometimes in stormy waters, these ideas are presented while trying to steer honestly and on course. Like Steinbeck's boat, which has shaped the human mind and soul, the feelings that identify with this boat are deep and soul shaped, following almost 30 years of my work and travel as a nursing theorist.

Time and again during my career I have found that my concerns about nursing and the sacred caring–healing practices and traditions are not mine alone; they are the concerns and passion of nurses and women all over the world who share in this awakening of the human consciousness.

At one level, this work is a continuation of my earlier 'theoretical' works. At another level, it is beyond theory and beyond method: dare I say it, beyond nursing. It conveys a framework of both praxis and theory. The

Greek word 'theorem' guides me; back to the 'seeing' concept, which means 'to keep one's gaze fixed upon something' as a way to describe some truths as a form of reflection and contemplation (Fay 1987).

Human and ecological suffering is common throughout the world and restoring caring and the ancient sacred feminine has become a global issue; the sacred feminine that nursing symbolizes has been wounded and is in need of healing. Across the globe, nurses are committed to recovering the soul of nursing as a healing gift for our time. A different cosmology of transpersonal caring is posited here as a path for a new model to potentiate healing and to move us from the modern to the postmodern and beyond. Nightingale, and her timeless and enduring ideas and directions for nursing and beyond nursing, provides a template for further consideration for all health care providers.

As part of this book, I attempt to bring continuity, together with a new seeing and understanding of Nightingale within a postmodern context that takes us into the 21st century and the new millennium. Metaphorically, nursing can relight the lamp and light of nursing's past calling and ethical commitments, within a broader context of advanced caring–healing praxis while framed within a unitary, 21st century cosmology.

This book is to help me, other nurses and the public to remember, rediscover and understand that the feminine caring–healing energy of nursing, as sacred archetype, can be a hopeful, and hoped for, paradigm for a new/old cosmology for health care and healing, so necessary at this point in human history.

Nursing is presented as a paradigm case for women and the caring–healing dimensions of nursing's work, work that has been expunged from the traditional Western world cosmology, and particularly the modern masculine archetype of traditional science and medicine—the latent, and not so latent, archetype under which nursing has located itself within this modern era of the 20th century.

The theory part of this book is related to seeing within a new cosmological view of reality, describing some ancient but new scientific truths and worldview shifts, and helping to keep our gaze fixed upon the purpose of our 'being', our so-called 'calling' into caring–healing work.

Finally, I write now from a position in which I face myself and my own truth about nursing in the world, from one century to the next. I write to find a different voice, to call forth my own spirit, beyond my socialization and professionalization into what has been called 'patriarchal anthropocentrism' ('man-centered or human centeredness') (Fox 1991, p. xi). I write for anyone 'trying to fashion a world that will hold all the people, all the faces, all the Adams and Eves'.

Hearing

Nurses around the world have told me that the Center for Human Caring in Colorado (now being expanded to be an International Center for Integrative Caring Practices), which I helped to establish in 1986, symbolizes a place that holds the light for nursing's transformation. This book, consistent with the Center's work, can be seen as an attempt to exercise conscious responsibility toward helping to bring about a genuinely new epoch in nursing's history, consistent with a transformative consciousness occurring around the globe—a non-linear jump from the modern to the postmodern and beyond.

As with my other works, this book also concerns itself with metaphysics in that it encompasses consideration of both ontology and epistemology of caring and caring consciousness in relation to a caring–healing praxis. It concerns itself with concepts which are neither clearly defined nor definable, nor is their meaning accessible through the type of modern, linear, rationalist analysis associated with the modern tradition of both medical and nursing science. It goes beyond what we normally regard as empirical factors and the material world and embraces mind, consciousness, soul, the sacred, the ancient and contemporary Yin emergence.

You will see how I am influenced by quantum science views, holographic notions, arts and humanities, poetry and metaphor as well as traditional science to help demonstrate an expanded view of person, humankind and of transpersonal caring. Here lies a paradox in promoting a fully embodied spirit (in the personal, expanded notion of what being human means), while also transcending the personal and generating concentric circles reaching from the innermost point to the universe (and vice versa).

We recognize that, even though medicine and other health professions throughout time have been based upon a philosophy of caring and healing, we find ourselves at the end of the 20th century having to make a case for caring and healing. Of course we all benefit from the rise of modern medicine, with its scientism, its flourishing biotechnological cure successes. Even as we face the next century, mainstream medical science will continue to rely on its biological science foundation and breakthroughs for its future, as perhaps it should. But at another level, modern medical science and the entire system and culture in which Western medicine is located are in chaos and crisis. It is an era that Smith (1982) refers to as 'postmodern', an era and accompanying mindset that Heidegger (1971) and others note is seen as a work, not of art, but of technology. It is an age that has become value free and is characterized by its shapelessness in that, while it lacks definition, it clearly rules out and delegitimizes values and existential meanings (Smith 1982). It is a time when the soul has ceased to exist in the modern mind (Griffin 1992, p. 50). During this modern time, we have come to think of a human being as a kind of machine, or as a cog in the greater mechanism of society, operating within another machine, the earth, which operates within the greater mechanical design of the universe (Griffin 1992, p. 50).

The modern/postmodern juncture is characterized by a loss of faith in any higher order other than human order and control (Smith 1982). Smith (1982, p. xii) further describes this turmoil of time between thought systems and an era of 'in-between': 'It is as if, standing before a picture window that opens onto an alpine landscape, we have lowered the shade to the point where we can now see little more than the ground at our feet'.

As Lewis Mumford (1970) pointed out, we are at a critical juncture as we enter into a new century. He emphasized that while change is always taking place, there are particular periods when society goes through a more fundamental kind of change, involving all its institutions and the basic aspects of its culture. The dominant assumptions of society are irrevocably changing. In Smith's eyes:

> In the perspective of history, the latter part of the 20th century is likely to rank with the 4th century, which witnessed the triumph of Christianity, and the 17th century, which signaled the dawn of modern science, as one of the very few that have instigated genuinely new epochs in human thought.
>
> (Smith 1982, p. 4)

During such a dramatic time in human history, we are called upon to revise the very foundation of our so-called modern assumptions and ideology about science and medicine, caring and healing, and about the deeper meanings of masculine–feminine. Mumford (1970, p. 9) reminds us that during historical periods of major transitions, 'every transformation of man (sic) ... has rested on a new metaphysical and ideological base; or rather, upon deep ... intuitions ... whose expression takes the form of a new picture of the nature of man (and woman)'.

Aberdene & Naisbitt (1992, p. 16) predict that 'the most exciting breakthrough of the 20th century will occur, not because of technology, but because of an expanding concept of what it means to be human'. Harman (1991) calls this turn the 'second Copernican revolution', the first being a revolution of the outer world, the second a revolution of the inner world, of human consciousness.

It is timely and appropriate that the leadership for problem solving these deeply rooted matters of Western thinking will, and should, come from the medical, nursing and health professions. Human thought akin to Mumford's metaphysical and ideological shift can result in a transformation of health care as we know it, as well as in a transformation of professional education and practices. Redefining nursing within a deeper archetypal model which reconnects mind, body and spirit will help us to remember our evolving consciousness, our human–environment–nature–cosmos connection of the past, present and future. This perspective will provide a new ground of meaning and being-in-the-world, and will break through into a new world-view, for another time.

This next turn in nursing and Western society's evolution is a turn toward a restoration of and reverence for the sacred, for the soul, and for wholeness and completion. This will come from reconnecting with the archetypal feminine energy, of which nursing has an abundance. However, this archetypal dimension of nursing has not been actualized; indeed, it has been repressed and distorted during this century.

The excitement is that this perspective is now awakening in the human consciousness, from within and without. It is part of, and central to, the emerging disciplinary paradigm of nursing qua nursing within the postmodern era, in contrast to the modern evolution of nursing qua medicine.

Caring in nursing conveys body physical acts, but embraces the mind-bodyspirit as it reclaims the embodied spirit as the focus of its attention. It suggests a methodology, through both art and aesthetics, of *being* as well as *knowing* and *doing*. It concerns itself with the art of being human. It calls forth from the practitioner an authentic presencing of being in the caring moment, carrying an intentional caring–healing consciousness. It concerns itself with the transpersonal and transcultural, and with the objective, subjective and the intersubjective. There is openness to another possibility of being in the world, with caring and healing as a global ontology within an expanding cosmology.

Without clarifying and changing our cosmology—that which teaches us to behold the awe and terror of the universe—'our world is too small; if our worlds are too small, so too are our souls' (Fox 1991, p. 149). In *the era of today*, our souls are too small as a result of the human-centeredness of the universe and of our civilizations.

Our cosmology is one way through which we can enlarge our souls during *this postmodern era of crisis* in the human condition. Matthew Fox believes our cosmology is the corrective to the myopic worldview and will help us to re-experience the awe, divinity, reverence, sacred gifts and blessings of the universe: to rediscover radiance and beauty. It is a time to honor our being here and to honor one another and all living things. One such cosmology is related to caring at the human and cosmological level since one reflects the other, but only if located within a postmodern cosmology that takes us beyond the modern toward another relationship with ourselves, and planet Earth and the divine.

Caring in nursing and among all health professionals requires both theory and praxis, moving beyond mere thinking to action, based within a cosmology which embraces critical reflection within a different framework, and creative choices of being within a caring–healing model. Caring theory assists in 'moments of seeing' (Fox 1991) within each caring moment, thereby transforming our being. It moves from seeing to being within a caring moment of possibility. This moment becomes open space, generating a new field, a new potentiality, which can lead to a new moment of action. Such an awareness can be a transformative moment of praxis, a concrete engagement with other(s) for a reflective, yet spontaneous, action which becomes transcendent.

Considering nursing as archetype is one way to help us see, and keep our gaze fixed upon, the sacred acts of caring–healing. Nursing becomes a metaphor for the sacred feminine archetypal energy, now critical to the healing needed in modern Western nursing and medicine.

Words of war, words of peace

Metaphors are not just the concern of the poet or the literary critic. They are not just figures of speech, but represent the ways in which many kinds of discourses are structured, and powerfully influence how we conceive things (Sarup 1988). It may be tempting to consider metaphor as illusory, soft and even trivial; it is easy to dismiss as unscientific or non-rational a mere substitute for the hard analysis that rigorous thought requires. But it is clear that metaphor belongs as much to philosophy and science as to poetry. The act of thought and science itself are inseparable from metaphor (Watson 1987, p. 10).

We see how our ordinary scientific, medical and health languages are in part structured, understood, performed and talked about in terms of war. Words become weapons. There is a position to be established, and defended; you win or lose. You have an opponent, whether it be an idea, a person, a disease, or even life itself, with which you do battle, attacking to destroy, defeat, conquer and win. We intercept ideas rather than intersect with ideas (Sarup 1988). We separate ideas from each other, rather than connecting them; we strive to control our environment and nature rather than living in harmony and balance within it. This has been the century where metaphors of war, violence, control and greed became prevalent throughout the social, health and political fabric of individuals, communities, businesses and the highest political offices.

It is through such metaphors that we have shaped our field of modern thought and action. It is important that the metaphors we employ or accept are made explicit so that we may better understand how they affect our seeing and being. They can be helpful or destructive. They can promote unexpected or subtle parallels or analogies. They can encapsulate and put forward proposals for another way of looking at our reality or a given phenomenon.

Tarnas (1993) indicated that the human condition and human experience itself, while established by a multitude of concrete biological and historical factors, is shaped also by transcendent, universal, spiritual and metaphysical patterns or modes of experience; archetypal and metaphysical forms which continuously inform the elements of human experience into patterns and configurations. These transcendent, universal, spiritual and metaphysical patterns inform caring–healing practices in embodied and spirit-energy form. They connect and transcend simultaneously, permeating each experience and each worldview, consciously or unconsciously.

It is through nursing, as sacred feminine archetype, that I seek to encapsulate another life-generating metaphor of caring, healing and peace which counterbalances the dominant metaphors of war as the existing thought system of the 20th century. It is by remembering the archetype that ancient wisdoms and enduring truths are conveyed and through which tacit knowledge is expressed. As Fox (1991) said, it is Sophia, as dynamic, flowing, feminine energy archetype and metaphor, who brings wisdom; it is that which undergirds and permeates all things; it is She who brings order from chaos. It becomes both an object of intellectual pursuit and the fruit of awe and wonder. It is in Eros that we find rest, delight, joy and creation. Fox refers to Her as the way of the authentic. She defends the poor instead of upholding the powerful; she is co-creator of an on-going process of spirit in the universe; she teaches and gives birth to the sacred ways of living, being and healing; she is both prophet and spirit who returns us to wholeness and holiness. A new cosmology is contained within the sacred feminine archetype, one of transformation, whereby all things can be made new or whole (Fox 1991).

Reintegrating—archetypes

It is ironic, to say the least, that mainstream nursing during the 20th century has not understood this aspect of its work. Instead, it has identified for so long with the masculine archetype of modern medicine, the cosmology of patriarchal anthropocentrism (Fox 1991), that it has forgotten its origin. This has occurred often to its own confusion and to the detriment of its evolution and mission in trying to fashion a better world for caring and healing practices.

It is also more than ironic that nursing, as the largest female health profession in the world, has been marginalized, blamed, ignored, dismissed and labeled as 'part of the problem' in the current health care crisis. Mainstream discourse about health care reform has not identified nursing as one of the primary solutions.[2]

Due to nursing's history and internal crises, it has tried to obtain its power by aligning with the powerful other (masculine-medicine archetype). It has been ineffective in coming into its own, or seeing that it holds transformative solutions to the system crisis, not patchwork approaches that perpetuate the existing paradigm problems (see pp. 33–46 for a fuller discussion of nursing's internal problems).

To date, the voices for nursing's solutions remain largely within the modern Western cosmology; such a position takes nursing in the opposite direction from where healing and solutions can occur. Nurse as archetype and metaphor for woman and healer provides another, deeper dimension

---

[2] The exception is the nursing profession itself, with its own united position on health care reform. The problem is that its organized position has not been incorporated into mainstream thinking. It is not a consideration among the powerful medical, male-dominated approaches that are largely concentrated on medical services financing reform. This is not true health care reform, within the context considered here. The second problem is that the dominant reform debates are still located, even inside organized nursing, within the modern masculine archetypal model of medical care.
If nurses have anything to offer, it is proclaimed to be as primary care providers, under an umbrella term of 'physician substitutes', not within a mature nursing caring–healing model that can offer a transformed approach to health care.

to the 'nurse equals woman equals nurse' problem. Nurse and woman as healer, joined by compassionate, nurturing, intuitive, balanced men (nurses, doctors and others) can more fully actualize the whole medical healing system (Achterberg 1990). Caring and healing are about *relation*, not *separation*, about meaning, being and finding sacredness in the act of caring itself. This, in turn, becomes what Whitehead (1953) called the 'eternal now'—a timeless, transcendent moment for humankind.

As currently constituted, however, the idea of woman and nurse as healer is incongruent with the dominant medical science cosmology of allopathic practices: practices which both define what constitutes clinical practice and determine what matters and counts as reality. These dominant practices, at this moment at the turn of the 20th century—the century of the most advanced allopathic medical revolution in the history of humankind—have all but eliminated any sense of the sacred or the feminine healing dimensions from our so-called modern institutions of healing.

We all recognize that the Western cultural cosmology, while changing, still continues to endorse the hierarchy of men over women and therefore medicine over nursing (masculine archetype over feminine archetype), rather than promote the idea of two co-equal, flowing, intermingling energies needed to make a whole. Today we see (we have to see) that, to some extent, the modern cosmology for medicine and nursing is required to change and yield, as we all must yield, to what Toulmin (1990), like Smith (1982), refers to as the 'postmodern era': an era which lies within a different cosmology and worldview. Here we must operate from a place of possibilities of *what might be*, rather than accepting *what has been* and no longer works. Nursing, therefore, as the paradigm case for women and healing within an evolving worldview in search of the ancient sacred feminine, balance and harmony, can be seen, at best, as the single most promising event in health care (Achterberg 1990) and, at least, as a hopeful paradigm for a postmodern era and beyond.

For when we awaken from our lethargy and engage in contemporary progressive thinking, without being threatened by it, then perhaps we can admit to ourselves that it is the lack of a feminine viewpoint that is at the heart of the problem in American and Western medicine (Achterberg 1990, Remen 1994). When nursing's sacred feminine belief system and healing consciousness re-emerge and are expressed through professional practices, then the whole system can be healed.

First, however, nurses and nursing must heal themselves from a century of modern Western medical dominance which is embedded in a cosmology of masculine archetype supremacy.

My desire for writing this book is to bring about a deeper discourse within nursing and health care of the issues that are already evident. In tapping into this existing awareness, I write to find meaning and words to tell another cosmic story, one that comes through me across time. I write to hopefully provide myself and others with the courage to be true to one's 'calling' and all that conveys within the modern–postmodern turn and beyond. Part of this writing is to keep the voices of nursing accurate across time. I am one voice among millions. We each write or tell our stories about our work, to keep our voices active and accurate during a passing time in nursing and women's history at this turn of the century.

2

Moving from text to margin

....

Think of it as a page. The main text is central; it is the text of ... daily preoccupation and jobs, keeping things going. This text is negotiated mostly by convention, routine, habit, duty: we have very little choice in it. So long as we are in this text, we merely coincide with our ordinary selves ... the margin is the place for those feelings and intuitions which daily life doesn't have a place for and mostly seems to suppress.

(Donoghue 1983, p. 129)

The 'text' within the modern/postmodern discourse is the so-called 'master narrative', a narrative of power, control and domination of possibilities. This is what Foucault called 'normalization' of power, on which homogeneity and hegemony impose themselves, allowing people 'to determine levels, to fix specialties, and to render the differences useful by fitting them one to another' (Foucault 1984, p. 197).

The main text refers to that which is worthy or respectable. Most commonly, what is worthy or respectable is identified with white, middle-class values, for so long taken for granted as 'American' (Greene 1991). As a result of having been taken for granted, these values have to be named, examined and critiqued as part of an awakening of the human consciousness. This awakening allows us to see that which is not in the text, as well as that which is included: to disclose that which is missing and to make visible that which is rendered invisible. Thinking in the postmodern era and beyond is about considering the *margin* in addition to the *master text*.

The margin is where things happen beyond what is and where we move to spaces where we can create visions of other ways of being and ponder what it might signify to realize them. To move into those spaces or clearings requires a willingness to resist the forces that press people into passivity and bland acquiescence. To resist such tendencies is to become aware of the ways in which certain dominant social (and professional) practices enclose us in molds or frames, define us in accord with extrinsic demands, discourage us from going beyond ourselves, from acting on possibility … and to be less likely to confine oneself to the 'main text' (Greene 1991, p. 28).

The medically dominant *text* of medicine and nursing is embedded in the hierarchical structure of the power/knowledge nexus of medical science, the medical profession, and its 'expert knowledge' claims about the human body, disease and illness. This expert knowledge has empowered it to diagnose, treat and 'normalize' the human experience of health and illness to medical knowledge and practices. Nevertheless, both medical and professional critiques[1] in recent years have come under increasing criticism for being uncaring, stigmatizing, and disempowering (Mitchell 1996, p. 201).

The *margin* is where nursing's imbedded practices are being uncovered and where they differ from the medical text. It is in the margin that we seek to disclose a subtext which, in turn, creates a clearing for a new text that goes beyond the modern/postmodern discourse, and opens up new vistas of being in the world, perceiving new patterns and possibilities for caring and healing of self, other and life itself.

---

[1] This critique from the public is related to the rise of corporate-industrialized medicine in Western nations, and USA health maintenance organizations, which have forced professionals to use cost as the driving forces for care decisions, often to the exclusion of the inner healing needs of individuals.

In this emancipatory clearing for nursing and all health care practitioners, there is another movement towards the making of some common world: a world in which individuals and practice communities transcend traditional professional boundaries and come together to share unabashed love for caring and healing practices, integrating the human–nature–universe relationships in artful, aesthetic, healing practices and bringing together art, science and spirituality to a new depth for those engaged in healing work.

This book is organized into texts and margins that weave in and out of the pages, ultimately leading to a transformed perspective for nursing and caring–healing work—a perspective which is beyond the postmodern.

Deconstructing and reconstructing

Deconstructing

Deconstructing can be defined as:

> *To attempt to locate the promising marginal text, to disclose the undecidable moment, to pry it loose ... to reverse the resident hierarchy, only to displace it (transform); to dismantle in order to reconstitute what is always already inscribed.*

> (Derrida 1976, p. xxvii)

In this instance, the privileged term (medicine/curing) depends for its identity on excluding the other (nursing/caring), thus demonstrating that caring really belongs to the subordinate term (nursing). When one deconstructs the dominant term medicine/curing, which is foreground, and introduces nursing/caring, then there is a foreground–background shift. If nursing/caring becomes the foreground, then medicine as foreground dissolves into the background.

According to Derrida, the first move in deconstructing is to overthrow or dismantle the hierarchy. The next phase must thus displace this hierarchy. Here, in this text, we see that the nursing/caring/healing model has already been acknowledged as a model to replace the resident dominant hierarchy.

Numerous nursing authors and the public are positing such a reversal; there is widespread disillusionment with the dominant, modern medical system.

In the postmodern deconstruction/reconstruction framework, curing and caring become inverted, and caring and healing relationships and practices become the highest level of commitment that health professionals can make to self, other and to humankind, as well as to the planet Earth (Gadow 1988, Watson 1988a). In other words, within our Western world-science mindset, we are being asked to change certain habits of mind. We are being reminded that the authority of medical cure is provisional.

Modern nursing has operated from the margin of the dominant cure model. Within the modern world of nursing, invisible concepts such as caring, comforting, compassion, physical caring, supporting, relationships and feminine healing energy already reside unnamed in the gap between the terms 'medicine' and 'nursing'. The caring, health and healing concepts and practices from nursing's most ancient and contemporary practices are already inscribed, even though they are invisible and have been demoted. In nursing in the postmodern era, the marginal caring–healing practices, which lie in the gap between modern medicine and modern nursing, shift from the margin to the center. Those marginalized caring–healing practices become central and harmonious within the postmodern era and beyond. Medical cure becomes background to the caring–healing foreground; this new foreground becomes an integrating framework for the whole system. The postmodern inversion of the 'resident hierarchy' of medicine is as necessary for medicine as it is for nursing, returning both medicine and nursing to the centrality of their caring–healing–health practices.

As futurists remind us, postmodern deconstruction/reconstruction is already a part of the human condition and is, in part, a preparation for a new type of society (Sarup 1988, p. 118). The knowledge hierarchy and power within the postmodern era cannot survive unchanged, and are simply two aspects of the same question: 'Who decides what knowledge is? Who knows what needs to be decided?' (Sarup 1988, p. 119). As Sarup framed it, the postmodern discourse involves a critique of metaphysics, of concepts of causality, of identity, of the subject and of truth (p. 4).

This discourse about the critique of the modern against the ambivalence and uncertainties that are constantly questioned within the postmodern runs across and revisits all the issues between medicine and nursing, and between masculine and feminine energy as archetypes for human existence. Each of these issues is now being deconstructed and is awaiting reconstruction. The deconstruction of the dominant modern 'center' is emerging in areas such as quantum physics, systems thinking, ecological concerns, feminism, existential phenomenological philosophy, critical social theory, human inquiry work, hermeneutic interpretative inquiry, and postpositivist thinking.

The shift developed in this book is greater than just a *paradigm* shift, and goes beyond modern/postmodern thinking toward a deep *ontological* shift, transforming our very being and requiring us to reconsider what it means to be human. This ontological shift invites us to recognize the evolving human potential that is emerging from the most recent 20th century phenomena whereby there now exists a symbiotic relationship between humankind–technology–nature and the universe. As we shift our gaze from the conditions of modernity to those of postmodernity and beyond, we enter into an era that requires a transformation of everything we thought we knew and tried to work toward within the modern era of health care (Watson 1989). However, underlining all the latest developments within postmodern thinking, there lies a timeless ethic of caring and an honoring of the centrality of caring–healing relationships. They have to be considered anew within an expanding model that incorporates the ontological shift required.

Reconstructing

Reconstructing is to move the caring model from the margin and to disclose nursing as the 'holding space' for the emergence of the sacred feminine archetypal healing energy; to pry it loose; to reverse the resident hierarchy, only to displace it (transform it). It is to dismantle, ethically and scientifically, in order to reconstitute what is already inscribed on the margin. Nursing becomes both metaphor and dynamic archetype for a caring–healing model for all health practitioners in the next millennium. The model is grounded in nursing's marginal text, but when brought from the margin to create a new center, the model simultaneously transcends nursing, becoming transdisciplinary and serving as a blueprint for 21st century thinking.

3

In search of the sacred feminine: voices from the margins

All transformations begin and end with self.   (Mumford 1970, p. 420)

Dreaming

The Aborigines of Australia have a saying. They say that the white man/woman always follows the road that is paved. In the Aboriginal world, they have another way. It is through dreamtime. Rather than follow the road that is already paved (and in this case already crumbled and broken), they throw the road out ahead of them and dream it up. The dream described in the journal entry here helped me to see the relationship between my dream and my dreaming of another way that is deeply rooted in the arche-type of human existence and the deep psyche of the mind.

Journal entry
Tuesday, December 22, 1992
Boulder

I had a superb dream about 3 nights ago that I'm just now catching up on. I was at an international, formal event and in the midst of social–professional protocols and so on, with a long ceremony which was to follow with more social interaction. I saw and greeted a few international friends from the UK who were very cordial and pleasant. At this time, I really didn't want to stay for a full blown social–professional ceremony, but felt obligated to do so. Then one of the women looked at me and said 'but you might have to share a room' and I thought to myself, I really don't want to share a room. If I do have to share though, I hope Doug is here to share with. I really wanted to have the freedom to leave, but I did not know my way out. Then I was drawn to a small child, a boy of about 8 or so, who led me down into the labyrinth of the building (a long narrow corridor) to get me to where I was supposed to go. I didn't want to go where he was leading because it led through old, sterile, institutional halls and a hospital basement-like setting. I said out loud (in the dream) 'I don't want to be here.' The child led me gently and lithely onward. Finally, I said 'how do you get out of here?' By now I was speaking to an old man whom I had seen off in the distance through the dim, musky corridor as we continued down this inner path, with its interior of dirt-packed floors and tunneled-out dirt walls. Now, suddenly, the boy had led me right up to this old, white-robed man. He was standing before a cave-like opening in the side of the earthen wall and was now climbing through this to the other side. Just as he did so he pointed forward with his left arm outstretched so that I could look inside the cave. Then he pointed to the left

Perhaps one of the greatest tasks for postmodern nursing and beyond is for nursing to heal its estrangement from the sacred feminine creative energy, which would not only help nursing to heal itself, but would also help to heal the unbalanced medical system and the culture of this time. My dream somehow represents this revelation, at a very deep level, with regard to my own personal work and journey toward discovering, exploring, trusting and connecting with my inner self. It is also a message to myself and to others that the real work of caring and healing starts with self, and only from there can transformation occur.

In following an inner path toward the light, Heidegger (1971, p. 53) talks about how things happen beyond what is, when an open place appears: 'there is a clearing … a 'lighting' reaching beyond what we are sure we know'. Maxine Greene reminds us, within the postmodern perspective of the texts and margins of life, that it is often this invisible world, which for generations has been ignored, which enables us to engage authentically and adventurously with life and work. It is in this world that we may unexpectedly perceive patterns and structures in the surrounding world that we never knew existed. The curtain of inattentiveness pulls apart and reveals a completely new and different reality (Greene 1991). In the words of Marcuse (1977, p. 72), it is this world of the inner life, often accessible only through dreams, altered experiences or through the arts, that 'breaks open a dimension inaccessible to other experience, a dimension in which human beings, nature, and things no longer stand under the law of the established reality principle.' It is in this space, when people are released to attend and let their energies flow, that one can 'make perceptible, visible, and audible that which is no longer, or not yet, perceived, said, and heard in everyday life.'

As nursing honors its unity of being and its feminine life-giving energy, it heals the split within and without. As nursing takes responsibility for itself in a new way, it is reminding people of their wholeness, their origin and the necessity to honor life processes and creative energies and to preserve both life on Earth and Earth itself. It is here, with the realignment of the feminine and masculine energy of the universe and the reintegration of science, art, spirituality, physics and metaphysics, that we see again, as if for the first time, what is all

side of this inner room where I could see a narrow, winding, earthen staircase moving up toward another small opening of light leading outside. He then said 'there is how you get out.'

'Oh', I said, so relieved that I could see my path out—at the end there was a bright light leading to sunshine and out-of-doors. After seeing the light, the stairs and the way out I climbed into the cave to make my journey but, in so doing, my eyes adjusted to the cave's darkness and revealed an interior world of beauty and magnificence before me. Then I heard the sounds of chanting and drums from the ancient Mayan–Aztecs in Mexico. There, to the front, was an earthen altar, golden, round and raised like a giant mushroom stool; there was also a crescent-shaped theater of seats, again, raised stools, mushroom-shaped, with a golden, earth-tone luster. I was transfixed upon seeing the joyous and sacred setting and hearing the ancient chants. I said to myself, 'Oh, I'll never again be a disbeliever about the sacredness of the earth, the inner core of golden light, beauty and sounds.'

I then talked with the boy guide and told him I wanted to go into this golden area to look at it and experience it more closely (it was safe now that I could see my way out). So we went up closer to the big golden stage-altar and there on the altar were all kinds of sacrifices: jewelry, flowers, silver, gold, little hearts on chains, and personal items people had given to honor the sacred. I knew I had to give something and looked at my rings. I thought about my turquoise rings, but I would disappoint D who had given them to me; my other silver frog ring seemed too small and insignificant and, while precious to me, was bent.

So I then considered my three-silver-circled ring that I wear on the middle finger of my right hand—the ring my dear friend E had given to me. I thought 'that's the one I'll give. E will understand, so it's okay.' I took off the ring and placed in on the altar with the others ... I then decided I was ready to leave, up the stairs to the left, following the light with a new sense of wonder, beauty, humility, honor and sacredness of the experience and the inner world. The boy and I then left and I awoke.

around us yet is invisible to the mind that has only adopted the master narrative text of the modern time.

Yet in the new century and new millennium, it is time to look *through* the window of the outer actual world, to bring 'as/ifs' into being in our experience and our daily being (Greene 1991). This could be a healing time when nursing and all health professionals understand that when persons are released to attend and let their energies flow, when we refuse to perpetuate the habitual separations of the subjective from the objective, the inside from the outside, appearances from reality, the margin from the text, that is when imagination and creativity create a new order and transformation in our daily lives, bringing what Virginia Woolf (1976, p. 72) called 'the severed pieces together'.

Nurses and nursing, in attending to this aspect of reality and human existence, can be part of the transformation that is required for the next century. This too is postmodern nursing and beyond. To reconnect nurse and woman in a deep, archetypal, healing feminine energy sense, read the following excerpts from Murdock's work and imagine the word 'nurses' at the start of each section:

Women are weavers, we intertwine with men, children, and each other to protect the web of life.

Women are creators, we birth young ones and birth our dreams (towards healing, wholeness, peace).

Women are healers; we know the mysteries of the body, blood, and spirit because they are one and the same.

Women are lovers, we joyfully embrace each other, men, children, animals, trees, listening with our hearts to their triumphs and sorrows.

Women are alchemists, we uncover the roots of violence, destruction, and desecration of the feminine and transform cultural wounds.

Women are the protectors of the soul of the earth; we bring the darkness out of hiding and honor the unseen realms.

Women are divers; we move down into the mysteries where it is safe and wondrous and oozing with new life.

Women are singers, dancer, prophets, and poets; we ... help ourselves remember ... who we are as we journey through life.

(From 'The Heroine's Journey' by Maureen Murdock © 1990. Reprinted by arrangement with Shambhala Publications, Inc., Boston.)

Later journal entry:
I frankly feel very alone and isolated, but I am trying to see, to find my way, to be led. I am trying not to be too gloomy or down-hearted but to focus on strengths, positive aspects and new possibilities. I trust that the inner light will emerge in and through the institutional gloom and despair and that the inner chamber will hold golden treasures and sacred power, even though it means giving up my three-chambered ring. Somehow, the sacrifice of that trinity of silver rings seems significant and symbolic.

Still later journal entry:
Does the three-chambered ring symbolize the unity of all? The right-hand/left-hand meanings, the inner and outer worlds, finding beauty and sacredness in the inner world and following the light to find my way through the outer world? A young child and an old, robed man became my guides to the inner world.

Journal entry
April, 1993

Perhaps there comes a time in each woman's life, as well as the life of each nurse, when she or he is faced with a particular choice about the sacred feminine archetype as the ground of being. As Murdock (1990) puts it:

For one brief moment, month or year, (maybe during a moment of life's intense pain, dilemma, transitions, crises) s/he is given the opportunity to be in a situation, to assess it, and to ask, 'what ails me?' If the nurse has wittingly or unwittingly chosen the path of masculine medical archetype, s/he can stoically continue, fine-tuning or even fighting for identity, idealizing the breadth and width of power and control and prestige—acclaim in the world of modern medicine. Or s/he can integrate these learned skills and connect with the sacred feminine and healing wisdom of one's calling—the authentic ground of being. Such a choice allows one unity with opposites, to have a positive relationship with the inner masculine and inner feminine. The result is wholeness, healing at the archetypal mythological level, as well as at the personal–professional level.

Choosing to follow the inner light

The Yin is a way of seeing, a way of understanding the world, a way of formulating solutions, and a very powerful way of acting in the world. ... The access to the sacred requires us to see the world through feminine eyes, that we reclaim our feminine capacity, that we value the subjective, the intuitive, the qualitative, that we not focus only on the surfaces of things. (Remen 1994)

There is a void felt these days by women and men who suspect that their feminine nature has gone to hell. Wherever there is such a void, such a gap or wound agape, healing must be sought in the blood of the wound itself. So the female void cannot be cured by conjunction with the male, but rather by an internal conjunction, by an integration of its own parts, by a (remembering) or a putting back together. (Hall 1990, p. 1)

As women, nurses and feminine archetype-aware men know, things are out of order and those who are aware have a responsibility to bring about a healing in our systems and our culture during this era. As many writers today remind us, we are blind to the fact that we are out of balance. Nursing becomes a paradigm case for the gaping wounds which will not be (cannot be) healed by conjoining with the masculine archetype as the ground of its being. The history of medicine and nursing within the Western cosmology now instructs us that, as we have moved more and more into the realm of logos over Eros, of left brain over right, there has been an increasing sense of alienation from that inarticulate source of meaning and life nurturing that can be called the feminine, the Yin of life, the chalice, the Grail.

The left and right hand

The profession of nursing during the modern period has experienced the sadness and the loneliness of alienation, but we do not recognize that we are imbalanced within ourselves as well. We have also been caught up in critical, destructive, war-like battles of our own; we too are engaged in battles against illness, disease, even the human condition, which is often something to be overcome, rather than experienced.

The masculine archetype, symbolized by the right hand of modern medicine, is

It is an acceptance of both the masculine and feminine within and without as a dance toward healing and wholeness for all—a collective remembering of that which somewhere we have always known.

As this remembering and inner/outer healing occurs, nurses individually and collectively are contributing to a change in the consciousness on the planet from one of addiction to hierarchy, conflict and power dominance, to one that (once again) recognizes the need for relationship, connection, beauty, balance, dignity and peace.

POEM FOR THE LEFT AND RIGHT HAND

The left hand trails in the water
The right is tying knots
The right stitches a seam
The left sleeps in the silk.
The right eats;
The left listens under the table
The right sears;
The left wears the rings
The right wins, the right loses
The left holds the cards
The left strikes chords while the right runs,
runs up and down,
up and down,
And when the right can't sleep and travels
around the world
against the clock
The left is buried
Oh left hand, you're so quiet
Do you have children, a dog, mistresses, debts?
It is the right that buys the groceries,
shifts gears,
Runs for high office
Feeds the baby little silver spoonfuls
It is the right that grabs the knife
to hack off the left hand.
The left hand waits
A blind dog
Holding in its mouth the right's glove
The knife falls, clatters;
The left hand is the right's
Only chance.

(From Krysl M 1980, with permission.)

the idealized profession of the 20th century; it is the machismo archetype of power and dominion, perfection, critical judgment, control, unlimited avarice and demands for more and more accomplishments and gain. Nursing has been swept along in the 'blade and the sword' approach to its development, but is now realizing it has to heal itself and its own imbalance.

If nursing is to heal and is to be an expression of healing for self, other and the culture of our health systems, we need to make our wounds conscious. We are challenged to release the blind and unconscious who cling to the rigid, driven, critical, masculine archetype that controls our psyche and our practices. As we deny our sacred feminine we deny our feelings, body, mind and soul. As we deny our ground of being, we serve the inner and outer tyrant in ourselves and our culture (Murdock 1990, p. 158).

Healing is accepting and naming the nameless, unloved, invisible parts left unchecked. The challenge of nursing is to heal the archetypal sacred feminine. As it does so, it contributes to the healing of the world. This perspective and challenge is as true for wounded medicine as it is for the wounds of nursing. We are now beginning to recognize it at the deep archetypal level of understanding. It is at this level that we witness the wounds in our culture and professional systems. It has been an out-of-control archetypal wound that has lost its way and now has to return to the ancient instructions: *heal thyself*.

Many women, men, and the wider public along with medicine and nursing, are now needing to take heed, and are.

> Everyone is partly their ancestors; just as everyone is partly man and partly woman.   *(Woolf 1976)*

From the margin: 'The alchemist'

The alchemist is a magical story of Santiago, an Andalusian shepherd boy who travels in search of worldly treasure. On his journey he finds teachings strewn along life's path, teachings about the essential wisdom of listening to one's heart, learning to read the omens along the way, and above all, following one's dreams. Coelho (1998) tells the story:

> Your inner man and inner woman
> have been at war.
> They are both wounded,
> tired
> and in need of care.
> It is time
> to put down the sword
> that divides thee in two.
>
> *(Murdock 1990, p. 155)*

> *But the sheep had taught him something even more important; that there was a language in the world that everyone understood, a language the boy had used throughout his time .... It was the language of enthusiasm, of things accomplished with love and purpose and as part of a search for something believed in and desired (p. 64).*

> *Maybe he was also learning the universal language that deals with the past and present of all people. 'Hunches', his mother used to call them. The boy was beginning to understand that intuition is really a sudden immersion of the soul into the universal current of life, where the histories of all people are connected, and where we are able 'to know' everything, because it's all written there (p. 77).*

4

Deconstructing modern nursing

....

*If ever a profession had to contend with misunderstanding,
misrepresentation, antagonism and exploitation, it's nursing.*

(Parsons 1917)

*More than any other professional woman, the nurse is a metaphor
for all women.*

The nurse question is the woman question, pure and simple.

(Jones 1988)

From (outer) stereotype to (inner) archetype

Images of nursing

While acknowledging that there are men in nursing, the reality is that the
issues which concern nurses are women's issues, and vice versa (Lewenson
1996). The image and identity problems remain problems of *nursing* and
females (Muff 1982, 1988). Nursing is still viewed as traditional woman's
work, but is done in a traditional man's world.

Nursing within the modern era has become a stereotype for itself and
women in general. Many images of nurses in art, history and literature

across time are negative and spotlight, focus upon and telescope the problems of nurses and women. As such, they reflect the general stereotypes of both, from spiritual to earthy, from nurturing to castrating. These stereotypes of nurses and women also range from whore to nun, from the angelic, maternal figure to the witch, evil seductress and sorcerer, from the Madonna to the battle-ax.

Jones points out that it was no accident that when *Playboy* magazine decided for the first time in its history to run a cover using only a woman's face (instead of nude body), the face used was that of a nurse, identified by her nurse's cap (*Playboy*, November 1983, in: Jones 1988). Apart from Nightingale's lamp, the nursing uniform, cap and pin have been widely recognized as visual symbols of the profession. The erosion of standard professional nursing apparel, however, has led to confusion. While the archaic stereotype has been eliminated, the profession itself has yet to find an image with which to replace its original symbols. Consequently, nursing's original symbols remain set as a stereotype in nursing and in the public consciousness.

> From the standpoint of political theory (and action), women ... (and nurses) dwell in the 'ontological basement' outside and underneath the political structure (and the professional/academic structure).   (Martin 1994, p.38)

The notion of an ontological basement is reflected in the media stereotypes of nursing. These embedded stereotypes have been depicted in the media in six major ways (Muff 1988, p. 211):

- angel of mercy
- handmaiden to the physician
- woman in white
- sex symbol/idiot
- battle-ax
- torturer.

Other images include the starched spinster; cool, soothing hands; rough, probing hands; bedpan; ministrating; medicating; and bathing. Both Muff

(1988) and Kalisch & Kalisch (1982) report similar images and, based upon their critiques and interpretations of the media, suggest that, while all stereotypes project the image of nurses as females, none reflects the intelligence necessary for nursing. Indeed, nurses are commonly portrayed in traditional and obsolete roles which do not reflect the specialization, sophistication and autonomy of what modern nursing has become. The image is negative, confusing and inaccurate, and perpetuates stereotypes that are not easily erased from public consciousness.

Other factors which reinforce and perpetuate the embedded stereotypes are what Muff (1988) calls socialization and sexism. These issues need to be acknowledged to show how nurses themselves, and the profession of nursing, compound their own dilemmas. We also need to see how external forces interact to reinforce both from within and without. I find it helpful to reference Muff with respect to these matters because she is outside nursing and brings a broader perspective to the issues than nursing's interior critique of itself is able to do.

For example, Muff (1988) discovered how much nurses, and nursing itself have been overwhelmed, confused and divided during the 20th century. She has challenged nursing's own worldview by pointing out that nurses talk about *unity* among themselves, but their real desire is often translated to be *homogeneity*.

Reverby (1987), also outside nursing, commented that nurses are still searching for a way to forge a link between their desire for altruism and their desire for autonomy. In other words, they are searching for the way to care in a society that refuses to value caring, and the way to serve without being subservient. Part of the worldview for nursing is based on the mores of Victorian times and what Smith-Rosenberg (1975) called 'homosocial networks' which served to overcome many of the limits of the cultural division of that time. Reverby (1987) indicated that this separate but unequal arrangement, combined with different visions for nursing within the nursing leadership, contributed to nursing becoming increasingly defensive and turning on its own rank and file. With this historical pattern, she observed that nursing continues to struggle to obtain the freedom to claim rights even to care or to differ. In many ways, little has changed.

Muff cautioned us that the issue for nursing is not one of disagreeing per se, but the fact that disagreement is interfering with nursing's progress. Nursing continues to have what Sartre (1963) and Laing (1965) referred to as 'ontological insecurity' about who and what nursing is or should be. It continually engages in internal debates about its status, its worth and its right to care and be autonomous. There continues to be a lack of consciousness and awakening to the impact of nursing's own forces within and without. There is also an acceptance within the profession, and by individual members, of how nursing perpetuates its own self-imposed restrictions, rather than finding its own voice.

Muff's work (1988) also highlighted the problems of socialization, isolationism, authoritarianism and perfectionism as part of nursing's responsibility. Nursing schools and nursing programs, for example, have a pattern and history of only admitting traditionally oriented women (i.e. oriented toward nurturing roles and natural mothering inclinations) into the profession. Historically, nursing education has been physically removed from mainstream education by social institutional forces, and this has not always been the fault of nursing. When liberated, however, the pattern of isolation remains, even to current times in mainstream academe.

Muff's critiques of nursing's self-imposed restrictions expose the use of jargon and esoteric language in its models and theories, which further contributes to the alienation of nurses from each other and from co-workers. She does not denigrate the need for theory but finds that the rigid, impractical, often arbitrary and even egocentric language used to describe theory has adversely affected nursing's image and isolation.

Authoritarianism has been a strong tradition throughout nursing's education and practice cultures and, to a lesser extent, of its research approaches. Muff (1988, p. 200) reminded us of how nursing instructors often believe (and teach) 'that there is only one right way to do things—their way!' Despite nursing faculty rhetoric about nurses being autonomous professionals, agents of change and leaders, faculty and institutions usually reward obedience and conformity rather than assertiveness, questioning and difference. Such authoritarian approaches stifle the creative, inquisitive, risk-taking behaviors necessary for a mature health profession.

Reverby (1987, p. 10) pointed out that little has changed over the years. Nursing is still divided over what counts as a nursing skill, how it is to be learned and whether a nurse's character can be measured by educational criteria.

Perfectionism is exhibited in the skills laboratories and the 'training' exercises of task performance, leading students to believe that only perfect practice is permissible in clinical areas. Muff (1988, p. 200) noted how even the safest most mundane chores are supervised: small details are invested with undue significance and danger. The 'life-and-death' nature of work is emphasized even if, in fact, some of it is 'boringly routine'.

A summary of the professional socialization imposed by nursing and its students is contained in the conflicting message passed on by nursing to each new generation: 'learn to be an autonomous professional, but follow the rules unquestioningly' (Muff 1988, p. 200). As any nurse or nursing student knows: 'nothing could be more crazy-making' (Muff 1988, p. 200).

Identity and boundary difficulties

In the steady continuum of history, we meet a divide between public and private events. Shifting from one to the other, the discourse changes. Even the tone of voices when entering the world we call private, slows down, drops a scale and perhaps softens.   (Griffin 1992, p. 33)

Nursing still struggles with the basis for and the value of caring (Reverby 1987, p. 10). One look at nursing's philosophies and theories reveals nursing as a liberating human science and human service, embedded in a caring context of relations, meaning and processes and committed to healing, wholeness, health and community. Another look at nursing and its texts and narratives reveals a limiting, traditionalist and rationalist power control model of itself and its means for advancing. As Reverby (1987, p. 10) put it: 'unable to find a way "to care with autonomy" and unable to separate caring from its valuing and basis, many nurses find themselves forced to abandon the effort to care, or [abandon] nursing altogether'.

Part of this dilemma and dissonance is caused by the obvious socialization and authoritarianism in the culture. Other aspects are self-imposed, some of which are related to nursing's developmental conflicts, and which contribute to the problems of stereotyping and image. Muff identified these as encompassing, both within and without:

- identity and boundary difficulties
- dependence/independence binds
- Nightingalism–Narcissism (self-esteem)
- greed and envy.

The identity and boundary dilemmas are manifest through the perpetual questions nurses ask of themselves, such as (Muff 1988):

- What is nursing?
- What is unique about nursing?
- What is not nursing?
- What are the boundaries between medicine and nursing?
- What are the boundaries between social work and nursing?
- What are the overlaps?
- What constitutes a profession?
- What constitutes a professional nurse?

The contemporary debate about identity and boundary involves the pressing questions of the moment, for example:

- What should be the required level of education for a nurse?
- What should be the required level of education for advanced nursing practice?
- What should be the required level of education for a nurse practitioner?
- What is advanced nursing practice?

Such questions have been running throughout nursing's past and current history. On the other side of the debate we find nursing establishing arbitrary models for nursing practice, creating false boundaries. Muff (1988, p. 202) uses the example of 'relabeling the problem-solving process … and calling it the "nursing process"—an exercise in creative writing, rather than theory building'.

Other aspects of the boundary issues with which all nurses can identify include the pattern of nurses at various times throughout the 20th century giving away major responsibility for nursing care to non-nurses, while taking on the discarded responsibilities of others (usually physicians or technicians). As Muff discovered by looking at nursing from the outside, nursing's roles and functions have usually altered in response to the needs of others, without a conscious decision by nurses to make changes. These changes have been made more by default than by design, and usually in response to changing medical or institutional needs.

As modern medicine became increasingly technical, nurses assumed many of the tasks that previously were within the physician's domain. These ranged from administering treatments, taking a blood pressure, doing a venepuncture and undertaking physical medical assessments, to assuming advanced practitioner roles within medicine's domain. Generally, nurses have been eager to take on these tasks, rarely questioning whether they enhance nursing, advance nursing's caring–healing practices or serve the public better. There has been limited attention to addressing questions about whether nurses' advanced medical skills assisted the physician and the institutional needs of the moment, or whether this so-called advanced practice assisted the public.

Such giving up and taking on of activities throughout nursing's history has left it and its public confused and uninformed as to what nursing is. Blind assumption of others' tasks has eclipsed the development of nursing qua nursing, which this book attempts to highlight for nursing's mature future.

This level of nursing's development has been referred to as the 'oyster-bed stage' of development where:

> ... *nurses were imbedded and cemented and struggled to survive, small shells of different levels of preparation and entry into practice clinging to a humped back, having the irregularity of something growing—the oyster shell symbolized by the fighting to have that place on the rock to which it fits itself perfectly and to which it clings tenaciously as it struggles to achieve a place.*
>
> (Watson 1987, p. 14)

The heart of the national debate at this moment is still located within the identity and boundary problems surrounding nursing, but important steps have been taken by the American Nurses' Association (ANA) to reconcile some of the historical dissonance in how nursing defines and redefines itself. For example, the ANA Definition and Social Policy Statement about nursing has been revised (American Nurses Association 1995) and offers a contemporary perspective to nursing's evolution and its view of itself. Attesting to the rapidly changing nature of nursing and its ongoing process of redefining itself, the final version of the ANA Social Policy Statement revised and expanded its definition of nursing, and reconciled the right hand/left hand dilemma discussed above, that is, the 'diagnosis and treatment' emphasis, rather than the

---

Box 4.1 Postscript to ANA definition.

Since 1980, nursing philosophy and practice have been influenced by a greater elaboration of the science of caring and its integration with the traditional knowledge base for diagnosis and treatment of human responses to health and illness. As such, definitions of nursing more frequently acknowledge four essential features of contemporary nursing practice:

- Attention to the full range of human experiences and responses to health and illness without restriction to a problem-focused orientation.
- Integration of objective data with knowledge gained to form an understanding of the patient's or group's subjective experience.
- Application of scientific knowledge to the processes of diagnosis and treatment.
- Provision of a caring relationship that facilitates health and healing.

(American Nurses Association 1995, p. 6)

---

caring–healing perspective. It is now a much more comprehensive definition than before (Box 4.1).

Part of the professional debate about the statement was whether (medicine's) 'power words' of 'diagnosis and treatment' were to be included in the revised definition. This issue became a source of almost unresolvable conflict, even though 'diagnosis and treatment' language, whether using a nursing or medical label, is rarely (and in many instances, never) used by hundreds, if not thousands, of nurses as they report on their practices (Tanner, personal communication 1995).

The ethics of nursing diagnosis have been critiqued by several nursing scholars, bringing to our attention the potential 'harm' and 'human suffering' created by the diagnostic process (Hagey & McDonough 1984, Harrington 1988, Mitchell 1991, Mitchell & Santopinto 1988, Shamansky & Yanni 1983). The diagnostic process and associated language require the nurse to assess, judge and label the thoughts, feelings and actions of other human beings, which in itself creates suffering related to feelings of being misunderstood, disconnected and alone. It leads to stereotyping, categorizing and objectifying humans and their lived experiences (Mitchell 1991). The aspects of control built into the diagnostic model is another ethical concern that has been noted by nurses.

Nurses acknowledge that diagnoses related to specific pathophysiological events are potentially least harmful in that they define a specific alteration rather than a judgment and labeling of human experience. The dilemma comes when the biophysiological alteration labels are mixed up with the labeling, depersonalizing, objectifying and controlling of human responses, experiences, health and even caring relationships (Hagey & McDonough 1984, Harrington 1988, Mitchell 1991, Watson 1989). It is at this point that the ethical dilemmas are most acute with respect to human suffering and potential harm. It is at this level that the biggest conflict regarding medicalization of caring processes, relationships and healing approaches occurs. It is also here that there is the greatest philosophical difference between a medical control/diagnostic language approach to nursing and a human experience model approach, with its centrality of caring–healing relationships.

The debate over language and power continues as constituted in the language of medicine, even though national and worldwide health care reform mandates are moving toward community-based models of caring and health preventive practices. Medicine is shifting from an exclusive emphasis on diagnosis to a concern with meaning and the subjective aspects of what the experience is for the person (ironically, the domain of nursing in its previous definition with its emphasis on human responses to actual or potential health problems). Could it be that as nursing once again takes on some discarded appendages of medicine, such as the technical diagnosis language, it becomes the medical technician, while medicine expands its boundary into complex caring–healing practices?

Similar boundary concerns were reflected in the 1993–1994 health care debate in the US. The emergence of the term 'advanced practice nurse' raised questions with regard to:

- Who can do it?
- What do they do?
- What is the necessary educational level?
- Are they practicing as medical substitutes or under a nursing qua nursing model of health and caring?
- Are they in a curing model without choosing it?

These and related problems haunt nursing, and are both self-inflicted and culturally and institutionally perpetuated. Dimensions of self-esteem, independence, dependence, greed and jealousy are further developed and discussed by Muff (1988). They are commonly known and experienced in nursing at all levels, whether admitted and made conscious or not.

Power inequities between medicine and nursing are so institutionalized that they are accepted as the norm. Muff labeled some of the selflessness in the concept of 'Nightingalism' as referring to both an undervaluing of self (and nursing and its feminine energy of caring and healing) and an overvaluing of others. As a result of these power inequities, nurses often cannot or do not express themselves and their needs directly. Reverby (1987, p. 10) suggested that nurses do not simply accept these power inequities as a result of their oppression, 'but because of some deep understanding of the limited promise of equality and autonomy in a health care system they see as flawed and harmful'.

Muff reported that nursing has its own myths about the adoption of roles such as victim, martyr and sacrifice being ennobling and even superior. The greed and envy she referred to is manifest in the lack of tolerance for diversity and differences, the desire for homogeneity and sameness, and the tendency to settle for the lowest common denominator for all, whether advocating education or practice roles. The slogan 'a nurse is a nurse is a nurse' is seemingly embedded in the patterns of being in nursing. We see examples of the competition and jealousy between diploma, associate degree, baccalaureate, nursing doctorate, nurse practitioner, advanced practice nurse and so on. Such built-in differences, within a culture that has institutionalized conformity and sameness, contribute to the constant horizontal violence in the field.

Nurses are well aware of the expression 'nurses are their own worst enemies'. There is rivalry for position, power, esteem and status, too often in the eyes of the medical establishment and institutional authorities, and even in the eyes of the public. These are examples of what Muff (1988, p. 213) referred to as 'identifying with the aggressor', thereby relinquishing nursing values (such as caring–healing) by aligning with those in power as a way to gain power. One of the core issues in the ANA national debate around nursing's revised definition is whether it should include the word *caring*. In the mid 1980s, during a nursing shortage, the ANA held a national public relations campaign carrying the slogan: 'If caring were enough, anyone could be a nurse'. This denigrated the caring attributes of the profession. An equally effective statement about nursing might have been: 'If medical science and technology were enough, anyone could be a nurse or doctor'.

The example of adopting terminology such as 'nursing diagnosis' as the taxonomy for nursing practice is another illustration of being co-opted by the language of powerful others as the way to attain one's own power. The rhetorical and existential question for organized nursing is: does such practice empower or disempower nursing, and what does nursing seek to accomplish through this approach—power for itself or human service for society?

The historical and contemporary socialization, professionalization, sexism and stereotyping of nursing, from within and from without, has stifled its development as a mature health profession with its own distinction and rights, capable of actualizing its own caring–healing values, knowledge and mature practices. In spite of these stereotypes and limitations, however, nursing has made great advances in education and practice, and is the largest single contributor to health care worldwide. Perhaps from the cultural images and historical journey of nursing we have a better idea of why nursing's contributions worldwide, and even nationally, largely go unrecognized by the system, the public and medicine.

Nursing continues to be seen as a backdrop against the dominant other. In the health care reform debates of the 1990s, it was cited as an economic drain on the system. Nursing care or salaries have been reduced or maintained at a low level as a means of containing costs. Meanwhile, the spending of millions of dollars on hospital expansions (even in cities that are 'over-bedded'), costly equipment purchases and perks for physicians have been defended (Muff 1988). In spite of the high profile of women's issues, insights and gains, physicians (largely male, although this is rapidly changing) are always positioned at the top of the pyramid in the hierarchical/patriarchal institutional culture of nursing's world.

Nevertheless, the nursing profession is at its strongest point at this turn in its history, and new modes are now available to it. A resultant question is whether nursing should consolidate, develop and enrich its new professional awareness and maturity *apart* from the current system or focus on analyzing and proposing changes *within* the current system (Thompson 1981, p. 222).

This book invites both options for consideration. Indeed, there is room for, and need for, both. Nursing can expand its existing role, continuing to make contributions to health care within the modern model by developing its foundational caring–healing and health strengths that have always been present on the margin. The other option, which nurses are rapidly undertaking, is for nursing to become a force for birthing an entirely new health and healing system of care, one that is more consistent with nursing's values and philosophy and which takes on a radically different dimension from that of modern nursing. The seeds for this new approach are contained within the book.

In the mean time, there is a continuing lack of public awareness of nursing and its diverse talents and contributions which, combined with nursing's internal confusion and debates, perpetuates and influences the status quo of nursing stereotypes. Even in the midst of nursing radically redefining itself for a postmodern practice and more, many of the modern nursing stereotypes are reinforced by the continued dominance of medical care (and nurses) by powerful male groups of physicians, hospital administrators and insurance companies. The change will come when nursing and nurses are directly aligned with the people they serve.

The pressing postmodern challenge for nursing

One of the most radical questions posed for modern/postmodern nursing has been put this way:

> *What will nursing be? What will nursing become? How will nursing be defined?*
> *... when the systems that have stood behind it and defined it, and given it its*
> *power, security, and employment, are no longer there? The systems either no longer*
> *stand behind nursing, or the systems no longer exist, due to the postmodern*
> *dismantling of such institutions. Then what will nursing be? Or become?*

(Moccia, personal communication 1996)

As we consider the postmodern turn in Western history and health care, nursing is poised to redefine itself from a nursing qua modern medical paradigm to reaffirm a nursing qua nursing postmodern paradigm, reclaiming its sacred feminine caring–healing archetype. Such a radical rethinking of the raison d'être of nursing is so necessary at this point in human and nursing's history. It requires a shift that moves from the modern, industrial, patriarchal framework to postmodern caring–healing practices. Such a shift will take nursing into the 21st century with the rights, autonomy, potential and power to transform itself and be co-creator with like-minded others to go beyond the Western medical mindset and become something else. Ironically, this 'something else' is already embedded and inscribed in the textual core and margin of nursing.

As Reverby (1987) reminds us, to achieve this, nurses will have to create a new political understanding for the basis of caring and find ways to gain the power to implement it. This shift creates space for practices within an equal partnership with other health professionals and the public, as opposed to a model of domination. It can be successful only to the extent that nursing redefines itself from the modern to the postmodern and beyond, while remembering its own ground of being.

The nursing profession, as it passes from the 20th to the 21st century, has to examine its identity, its boundaries, its maturity, its paradigms, its education and its practice models. At the turn of the century, poised between two worlds and times, nursing issues are like women's issues— issues which linger, unresolved, from one century to another, suspended and wedged between modern and postmodern dilemmas. Nursing, along with all other professions and disciplines, is witnessing the simultaneous peak and erosion of the Western culture cosmology.

To paraphrase Lather (1991), the question is: can nursing forget itself and become what it is destined to become, or must it remain part of the hegemony of a dissolving Western model of medicine and science? To transform and redefine itself for another time and cosmology, nursing must face some new truths about its power and possibilities. A new lens for seeing is one solution.

5

Seeing through Venus's mirror

....

Nursing has always been a much conflicted metaphor in our culture,
reflecting all the ambivalence we give to the meaning of womanhood.
Perhaps in the future it can give this metaphor and, ultimately, caring,
new value in all our lives.   (Reverby 1987, p. 11)

The crisis of modern (medicine/nursing) is the crisis of modern man.
                                                            (Tarnas 1993)

Not merely ... does nurse equal woman, but on an even profounder
mythological level, woman equals nurse.
                                           (Fiedler 1988, in: Jones 1988, p. xix)

The story of Venus's mirror

The myth and ancient story of Venus's mirror is about man and woman.
It is about the meanings we see reflected in the masculine and feminine
symbols used in the medical system of today.

The female symbol is a circle with a 'plus' under it and it is called
Venus's mirror (Fig. 5.1 left). When people relate to you from this feminine
side of themselves, what you see reflected in Venus's mirror is your own
strength, your own capacity, your own uniqueness (Remen 1994).

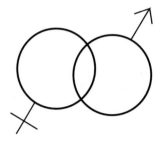

Figure 5.1 The 'mirror of Venus' and 'spear of Mars' symbols.

The other story is about the masculine symbol, the circle with the arrow on one side (Fig. 5.1 right). This is thought to represent Mars, the God of War, with his spear. When you have only the masculine style of system and health care, you feel the point of the arrow. You might be rescued, but the weapon is there to fight, to conquer (Remen 1994).

Nursing when considered as archetype and metaphor becomes the holder of Venus's mirror, collectively holding sacred space so the feminine energy and light can be reflected outward into systems of healing, into institutions and into our culture and world. By integrating Venus's archetypal meaning, nursing becomes a sacred mirror for inner healing. The archetypal image becomes a looking glass to see through the exclusive outer treatment (the 'fight and cure' approach) toward something deeper and more lasting.

In the deep archetypal sense that is intended here, the crisis of modern Western culture has been framed as the crisis of modern *man* (Tarnas 1989). In this archetypal sense, the crisis affects not only the evolution of humankind, but also manifests itself within our medical/nursing professions, our institutions and our healing systems.

From the archetypal perspective, Shepherd (1993), Tarnas (1989, 1993), Vaughn (1986), and many others reflect a historical position that the Western mind is running its modern course of evolution and has been almost overwhelmingly a masculine phenomenon: from Socrates, Plato and Aristotle, through Augustine, Aquinas, Luther, Copernicus, Galileo and Bacon, to Descartes, Newton, Locke, Hume, Kant, Darwin, Marx, Nietzsche and Freud. As Tarnas (1989) reflects, 'Most often a masculine gender word is used to refer to the collective human entity: anthropos, homo, homme, mensch, man'.

The Western intellectual tradition has been produced and canonized almost entirely by men, and has been informed mainly by the male perspective. In this modern, rational development of self and *man*, in our separating the mind from the body and the spirit and in dividing what is human from the primordial unity with nature, we have evolved to the rational, modern, human self. In so doing, the modern masculine mind has repressed the feminine, probably unconsciously, without intentionality, perhaps even out of necessity for our mature evolution. Nevertheless, at the archetypal level, and in relation to thinking and actions, the feminine energy has been all but expunged from the modern culture and cosmology. It becomes clearly manifest in the world of medicine and nursing.

Nursing and nurse symbolize, at this deep level, the repressed feminine. The contemporary conflict within the nursing profession is the conflict which exists in the archetypal consciousness at large. It is the repression of the feminine archetype among nurses and in organized nursing. This is evident in the ANA struggle with some nursing groups to retain the use of the terminology of 'diagnosis and treatment' as the power words to convey the control domain.

The alternative to nursing's defining itself vis à vis medicine is to define the natural, caring–healing, wholeness-oriented practices of nursing vis à vis nursing (in an archetypal feminine energy sense). The profession is confused and in conflict about how to resolve this issue. It is ironic that it is this one issue which has the potential to be *the* defining point for nursing's true identity, to take it past the modern stereotype, and flow into postmodern archetypal thinking and beyond. Essentially, if what Tarnas posits is true—the crisis of modern medicine is essentially a masculine crisis—it is understandable why nursing remains caught up in progressing within that archetypal consciousness.

The further irony for the nursing profession is that public consciousness and awakening have already foreshadowed nursing's awakening. The resolution, or antidote, which is already sought by the public to overcome the modern masculine crisis, which peaked in the 20th century, is the dynamic emergence of the feminine, redefining nursing from the modern stereotype within the masculine crisis framework to nursing's model of caring–healing within the sacred archetype. Such a redefining becomes an emerging paradigm for both men and women, for medicine and nursing as well as for the health care system in general.

In further clarifying nursing qua nursing (feminine archetype energy) we shift from war, control and power symbols, language and practices to the flowing feminine energy that taps life's natural processes and inner healing capacities for *self*, other(s), and all our relations with planet Earth and all forms of life and nature.

The public consciousness knows: there are overwhelming signs of feminine energy emerging that are consistent with nursing's archetypal meaning and maturing paradigm of nursing qua nursing. We see an increasing awareness of ecological issues and the embrace of the human community. Even our city blueprints and architecture have reflected the public disappointment with the incoherent picture we have formed, despite all our advances. This turmoil was reflected in an article on architecture by Herbert Inner, in the New York Times (1995), in which he wrote:

> *Urban Revisions', an exhibition of recent urban plans at the Museum of Contemporary Art in Los Angeles, offered a view of the city as a contemporary Tower of Babel, a metropolis abuse with the competing voices of modernists, post-modernists, en-traditionalists, deconstructionists, environmentalists and assorted mavericks. Consensus and solidarity were conspicuously absent.*

(Inner 1995)

He went on to ask: 'What kind of vision emerged from all these disparate urban revisions?' He suggested that the architectural profession now has a dawning awareness that the time has come to rethink some of the assumptions that have guided its thinking on urban issues for the past 30 years. He concluded his article with a rhetorical question: 'Has the century of progress been one grand march from hope to fear?'

The material world of architecture and social space has come to symbolize how the modern era has been recast in a self-image of separation and discord, resulting in what has been referred to as a 'well-intentioned, sprawling mess' (Muschamp 1995). This is in contrast to a comprehensive vision of a city of green, open space and a sense of place, where both bodies and souls may dwell.

All of this reflects part of the growing sympathy for non-Western and premodern, indigenous cultures. We are engaged in a widespread interest in mythological, archetypal, metaphoric and symbolic life meanings. In the University of Colorado, we, along with other disciplines, are seeking out phenomenology, hermeneutics, narrative, dialogue and the full range of non-objectivist epistemologies and methodologies to access the wholeness of human experiences and meaning.

There is a proliferation of mystical interpretations of modern physics: a reconnecting of the metaphysical with the material world of science. There is a linking of religion and science: an integration of secular and sacred. We are now tending to the soul and 'places for the soul.' Whether these patterns are conscious or unconscious, they have all become part of the postmodern exploration and are ongoing (Tarnas 1989, p. 25). Smith (1982) refers to this era of search as 'the postmodern mind', indicating that civilization is moving, and needing to move, 'beyond'.

The growing interest in a feminine perspective is evident in our material and non-material spiritual existence. We witness and participate in the renewed concern with the mystery of childbirth and in the dignity and sanctity of life processes including changing, growing, aging, dying, transcending and even *being*, breathing and the breath of life itself. Tarnas concludes that this dramatic development in human history, and in the passion of the Western mind, is not just a compensation, a surfacing of the repressed, but is a deeper, teleological (i.e. with an overall goal, or purpose) direction for the evolution, and some say the 'covolution' (co-evolution) (Briggs & Peat 1989), of the Western intellectual and spiritual being.

The deeper passion of the Western mind, according to Tarnas, is to reunite with the ground of its being ... to reconnect with the cosmos in a mature participation mystique. It is to surrender to the embrace of a larger unity that preserves human autonomy, while also transcending human alienation (Tarnas 1989). Jung (1989) framed this turn as a great shift in the contemporary psyche, a reconciliation between the two great polarities. It is a union of opposites (what has been called the sacred marriage in a universal sense) between the long-dominant but now alienated masculine, and the long-suppressed but now ascending feminine.

Nursing and medicine stand hand in hand as the paradigm for this dialectical reconciliation and movement. The solution and resolution are not for nursing to become more like masculine, archetypal medicine, but rather to more fully embrace and connect with its own sacred feminine archetypal source as the ground of its being. This returning and remembering the ground of its being is not to imply that nursing must give up all the technological and medical science knowledge and practices which have helped it to advance: the pendulum must not swing too far back the other way. It is rather an affirmation of the ideals and energy of the natural wholeness perspective that nursing qua nursing has to offer in the current medical world, which is largely devoid of the feminine and the sacred.

The emergence of nursing qua nursing, in the sense of a deep, feminine energy realignment, can not only result in a mature caring–healing profession, which nursing has always aspired to be, but can also allow nursing to transcend itself and be recognized as part of the larger whole. Each polarity requires the other for its fulfillment. The mature synthesis and metamorphosis of the nursing/medicine archetypal insights into caring, healing, treating and curing bring something fundamentally new. They bring an unexpected opening to a larger reality which cannot be grasped before it arrives, since this new reality is itself a creative act and part of the covolution process required (Tarnas 1989).

The danger of moving toward something fundamentally new is that nursing often becomes nervous about identifying with anything related to caring or feminine energy. It has, after all, worked so hard to prove its equality and power as part of modern Western medicine and science. The consequence is that if nursing does not emerge within its own paradigm—one that is qualitatively different but complementary to medicine—it will deny itself and its public those aspects that are now so critically being called for in today's curing systems. Denying the feminine archetype is to deny caring, relating, connecting, responding, intuiting, nurturing, feeling and cooperating. Yet these are all necessary to help resolve not only the modern/postmodern crisis of medicine, but also the crisis of humanity itself.

Once we consider nursing and medicine as paradigm cases for the change in Western culture, and see them release the hierarchical frameworks and practices that automatically rank one person, one profession, one race and one gender over another, then we can be free to see again. We can be open to value the wonder, beauty and benefits of diversity, pattern, process, multiplicity and creativity. We can be part of a movement toward wholeness and the healing of the deep wounds of Western civilization and the wounds of Western medicine and modern nursing.

The nursing/medicine archetypal representations in modern medical practices serve as both metaphor and exemplar of the crisis of our culture at this time. The postmodern changes emerging within these archetypal systems, rather than being seen as chaotic, can be seen as a source of ordering that carries hope for a new breakthrough for health care in its next stage of evolution.

As contemporary historians, scientists and philosophers remind us, this era awakens us to new facts as well as new meaning. It seems that the contemporary world is now beginning to recognize that *man*, and all that entails, is not the absolute fixed center of reality. This thinking can be seen as a fundamental metaphor for the entire modern worldview shift which is leading us past modern, Western assumptions into an emerging cosmology for a different world and a different century (Tarnas 1989). This thinking has to be something greater than just a paradigm shift. It is an archetypal, epochal shift in human consciousness—a fundamental ontological shift about what it means to be human—which is now allowing for an awakening and reuniting of the masculine and feminine, of curing and caring, and of the treating and healing principles and energies in our world, our countenance of being and our systems of healing.

Smith (1982) reminds us, however, that this change is still in process. We, the current generation of people and professionals, are playing a crucial but not as yet widely recognized part in the evolution. This epochal shift in the Western mind opens up a new level of discourse about modern medical systems and the caring–healing systems that are re-emerging from nursing's predominant, archetypal feminine principles, even if nursing or medicine as a system is not able to grasp it at this level. (Indeed, it seems to be some of the so-called 'alternative practitioners' who are giving birth to this dynamic, archetypal shift toward the feminine energy dimension of health care at this moment.) What seems to be happening is that some deeper level of meaning and natural processes are being uncovered and reinstigated, even though they remain marginal at the present time.

6

Deconstructing modern metaphors

....

Is the direction of any life (profession) inevitable? Or are there crossroads, points at which the direction might be changed?

(Griffin 1992, p. 130)

Have we truly outgrown war—war against ourselves, our bodies, our youth, our soul, our trees, ourselves? (Fox 1991, p. 9)

Modern medical practices became something of a war during the modern era, a war against disease, against the body and against the mind and spirit of humankind. This modern medical science revolution turned into a war for fame, greed, glory, control and domination. The modern medical war culture is laden with metaphors of fights, battles and conquests. It has become increasingly difficult to pursue the life-giving forces of caring, healing and peace against such masculine, archetypal adventures of war. The militaristic fighting mentality has permeated every social institution of our modern time, from the political to the criminal justice systems, to the child rearing, educational and research centers.

This modern cultural contamination of medicine and nursing, male and female stereotypes and archetypes, has generated and sustained a medical culture that obtains its stature from that which can be dominated and overcome. Its emphasis is solely on that which can be seen and touched, labeled and generally invaded. Such approaches are in sharp contrast to the latent archetypal traditions of women and healing.

Throughout nursing's history during this century, modern medicine (and subsequently nursing itself) worshipped the power of the blade and pushed away the life-giving feminine healing energy power. While nursing has always honored its inner power, it has been swept into the modern medicine revolution and ultimately has succumbed to the blade, denying its own development.

In many ways, the blade became the power metaphor for the modern, medical, masculine archetypal practices that medicine has become. Even within medical circles, the most powerful group in the hierarchy is often the surgeons. Medicine, in its out-of-control domination, has become somewhat like the blade of war. It is violent and war-like in its approach to the human body, assaulting and dominating disease and cure, life and death itself. This approach has little concern for the chalice of receptive, flowing, natural processes that harmonize and potentiate wholeness.

We see now where the blade in medicine is idealized and the chalice is undervalued. We also see how such a system is deeply flawed, out of balance and out of order. We see how the chalice/blade, partnership/dominator, feminine/masculine archetypal energies have had a profound effect on every one of our institutions and on our values. It is now affecting the direction of the evolution of medical–nursing professions and institutions.

Will our healing practices become more harmonizing and peaceful, or will we continue with our warlike approach? Will we promote, reward and prepare professionals for healing and wholeness, or perpetuate the domination of the blade model of medicine? Will we continue our emphasis on technologies that destroy and dominate in the name of healing, or shift to technologies and processes that sustain and enhance life, working with natural healing processes and the inner healer?

Regardless of the choices we make as professionals, the human evolutionary trend is toward a higher order, even in the midst of chaos. As Eisler (1987) and others (from physicists to chaos theorists) report, as we see power, greed, domination, war and oppression, there seems to be a human thrust toward truth, beauty, justice, harmony and wholeness. There is now a shift from the dominant Western science worldview to a search for the art of science (Briggs & Peat 1989).

Recent approaches in feminist and nursing scholarship, together with changes in physics and the philosophy of science itself, are examples of the introduction of a new, dynamic, different order and new patterns of possibilities in the midst of chaos. The current 'dominator' model (see p. 61) of modern medicine and nursing is, in large part, a consequence and symbol of a system that is breaking down.

An alternative to total *breakdown* is to *breakthrough* (Eisler 1987, p. xxiii), to find new ways for partnership models in medical and health care practices. This would balance the blade with the chalice, and allow a shift from the modern medical archetype dominating nursing and health care to postmodern thinking and beyond. Nursing and woman's feminine energy archetype model of caring–healing seeks to harmonize the whole.

Instead of medical virtues of toughness, aggression, dominance and control, can we bring forth values of caring, compassion, gentleness, love, mutual responsibility, natural life-giving and natural healing processes and practices? Such practices are dramatically different from those which have emerged during this time of Western cultural practices of mechanical medicine.

Each cultural era, whether prehistory, ancient, contemporary or futuristic, carries its distinct metaphors. The metaphors reflect the prevailing cosmology of the time. One symbolizes war, the other peace; one hierarchy, the other a cooperative circle; one the blade, the other the chalice; one the tangible seeing, the other seeing what is hidden, waiting to be revealed. Such a search for the intersection point of this time with the timeless requires another way of seeing.

Ancient wisdom/prehistory

In Lindburgh's writings in 1944, she describes looking down into the Mediterranean where she saw 'Crete like a pebble in a puddle, and all the blue mountains of Lebanon beyond'. The irony of her words in considering peace and war while looking over Crete is the fact that Eisler (1987) uses Crete as the exemplar of an archetypal feminine peaceful society and culture for another time in the prehistory of Western civilization.

> The adventures of peace should not and cannot be set up against the adventures of war.   *(Lindburgh 1944)*

Crete was the female ethos 'chalice' example. As Eisler (1987) reported, there has been no evidence of warfare in either the art or history of Crete. Achterberg (1990) targeted the Sumerian legacy to the healing arts, whereby for 2000 to 3000 years—until about 2600 BC—women were allowed to practice healing with little or no restriction and female occupations held great importance. In this culture, a woman was a reigning supreme deity who rejoiced with birth and whose body danced with the cycles of the moon (Achterberg 1990, p. 16). So woman, mortal and divine, was vested with healing mysteries and wisdom which carried the ebb and flow of life, and with peaceful existence. With such cultural healing practices, equal importance was placed on both the invisible and visible aspects of disease, treatment, curing and healing; there was an intersection of time with the timeless.

It was not only the cultures of Crete and Sumer which manifested a world and cultural cosmology that were not dominated by polarized separation and control of male over female. It has been reported that similar cultural models have existed in which the feminine life-giving creativity principles have been considered sacred and healing. This interpretation has been drawn from what is known through excavations of the art and culture of Minoan Cretan, Gnostic Christians, early Celts, Native Americans and Balinese, to name a few (Murdock 1990). Such traditions are also evident among indigenous cultures around the world, such as the Maoris of New Zealand, the native Hawaiian and American Indians, and the Aborigines of Australia.

Riane Eisler captures the feminine/masculine energies throughout her critique of art, history, religion and human society, past, present and future. Her metaphor of *The Chalice and the Blade* (1987) symbolizes the Yin-Yang differences and the two basic modes of society (or, in this case, the medical/nursing professional orientations): the dominator model and the partnership model. In the dominator model, referred to as either patriarchy or matriarchy, one half of humanity (or one medical profession) is ranked above the other. The partnership model is not based on hierarchical ranking but on connecting and linking. In a partnership model for medicine/nursing and health care, the archetypal energy differences need not be equated with either inferiority or superiority.

Eisler (1987) uses the prehistory of Western civilization as a tumultuous turning point for our cultural evolution. As she puts it: 'at this pivotal branching, the cultural evolution of societies that worshipped the life-generating and nurturing powers of the universe—in our time still symbolized by the ancient chalice or grail—was interrupted'. She refers archeologist Gimbutal who reported that the critical turn came about with the arrival of invaders who worshipped 'the lethal power of the blade'. This was the power to take rather than give life, the ultimate power to establish and enforce domination (Eisler 1987, p. xvii).

Fox (1991) listed the high point of the mystic prophets as the 12th century, when there were such teachers as Hildegard of Bingen, Francis of Assisi and Thomas Aquinas. Today there is again interest in old and new. There is a concern with seeking an antidote for the mechanized and

When I first read Susan Griffin's *A Chorus of Stones: the Private Life of War* (1992) I wanted to change the way I live my life, the way I work and write, and the way I relate to my ground of being.

She strung her words together so that they crossed time and space and, indeed, made a chorus from the silence of stones. Actually, Griffin, Dillard (1983) and indigenous folks alike remind us that the close study of stone will reveal traces of fire from thousands of years ago.

Many of us, and nurses in particular, are like stones, especially in matters related to caring, ethics, academe and science. Like stones, the history of nursing and of the medical and educational worlds are embedded in us. Like stones, nursing too carries a sorrow deep within and cannot weep or sing until that history is reflected.

Venus's mirror, a symbol for female, life-generating, healing energy and wisdom, which nursing carries as its covenant with the public across time, has been obscured, or at best has

non-mystical world, and there is a need for a bridge between the two. The current underside of history contains another story of war and peace captured by Susan Griffin in her book *A Chorus of Stones: the Private Life of War* (1992). (See the journal entry of April 1994.)

How do we prevent war? Woolf asks this question over and over again. Such haunting refrains of Nightingale and Woolf confront us with the political and philosophical question of ethical caring challenges and the imbalance of masculine and feminine principles, in our institutions in higher education, in our medical systems, in our society and in our world. Along with Woolf, should we too ask that our guinea (and vital energy) be spent in the cause of peace, not war?

Women also know war. The special writings of women, many of them nurses in the Vietnam war, in the book *Vision of War, Dreams of Peace* (Van de Vanter & Fuey 1991), demonstrate that women and nurses know war but seek peace.

They remind us of Florence Nightingale's experience of the horrors of war. The way she wrote over and over and over again the words: 'I can never forget'.

For centuries men have written about the glory of war; women too have gone to war, but have been dismissed as unimportant after the war is over (Van de Vanter & Fuey 1991, Preface).

In that same book, Norma Griffiths writes about the peace to end all wars:

Let us think no more
of the 'war to end all wars'
for only in complete destruction of all
would that be possible.
So let us think of the peace to end all wars
and perhaps
finally, working with the right tool
we can create the goal.

(Griffiths 1991, p. 201)

- -

The 7 deadly sins of male-dominated
society: capitalism, colonialism, communism,
militarism, urbanism and perverted uses of
biology and technology ... I reasoned that
the opposite pole to this in human terms is
the grandmother.   (Gahrton)

The question for this time, and perhaps for all time is: what should be the role of nursing, women, women scholars and indeed all scholars in the academic and professional community, in addressing the questions and ethical challenges with respect to caring and become a smoky mirror, during the modern era of medicine.

Compare the private life of nursing's caring with the public life of medicine. Compare the archetypal feminine of caring and peace with the masculinity of war, with war metaphors for living and dying, for systems, for society, for medicine and health care.

I return to Susan Griffin and wonder about the silent stones (the private life of nursing, of caring, of women and of the feminine) when considering caring ethics and models of healing that are embedded in nursing's feminine principles.

I cannot separate caring from peace in the world today. I cannot help but make associations between the feminine and caring and I cannot help but associate non-caring with violence and war, wherever it may be found, in the classrooms, operating rooms, battlefields and boardrooms. From one century to another, the questions and issues continue.

Griffin captured the connections and put it this way:

Teddy Roosevelt, or TR as he was affectionately known, became a symbol at the turn of the century for the revival of certain rough and ready masculine virtues ... he was the big game hunter, the cowboy, the statesman, who spoke softly and carried a big stick. He openly celebrated war. 'No triumph of peace could be quite so great (as war)' he said .... Peace, or the absence of war brought its own problems, among them, he warned 'the greatest danger being effeminate tendencies in young men'.

(Griffin 1992, p. 335).

Last year, a hotel in Boulder, Colorado (where I live) remodeled and renamed its popular restaurant after Teddy Roosevelt, complete with military mood and hunters' rifles and big game shrines of animals overhanging the gaslights and the new espresso bar. I cannot eat there anymore or even drink the espresso, which I love.

Last week, the University of Colorado Board of Regents rejected student-initiated health coverage for gay partners even though it was less costly than standard student coverage and was covered by student health fees.

How are we to untangle caring-ethics academic systems, nursing and scholars and the masculine/feminine energy realignment in our world? This question could be reframed: 'how do we prevent war, metaphorically, in our classrooms, our patient rooms, our board rooms, our pool rooms and our sports rooms? What *do* we as nurses in the academic and professional practice community have to offer to the project of preventing war, metaphorically and otherwise? How can we contribute to preserving caring, community and peace?

Such questions for us as individuals, and for our profession and academic and social community, are founded on an ethical commitment to human caring in instances where it is threatened individually, collectively, institutionally, or otherwise. Such questions are always before us, even when we consider who should enter professions such as nursing and education. Nursing and women (and now enlightened men) have the tremendous potential for enacting human capacities and moral activity in a society that is based on caring and peace rather than war. We are, nevertheless, still entombed in systems that place little value on such realities or interests, and indeed often place immense barriers in the path of such efforts.

Within the historical context of both Nightingale and Virginia Woolf, nursing and women could be posited as having a long history of deep struggles in the attempt to make and remake personal, private, professional and public space for the possibilities of enacting, or at least enabling, relationships for a caring ethic, rather than a fight ethic. Many in nursing, health science, and the broader academic community are aware of the caring theories and research in nursing science during the past three decades. Indeed, Leininger (1981) framed caring as nursing's central and underlying concept and essence.

Caring in nursing has been acknowledged as both process and intervention: as effect, as trait, as an ethical moral imperative, as an ontology and as a philosophical and scientific basis for nursing. This is a feminine perspective that helps to sustain humanity in the midst of cultural and scientific war mentalities against life and death. As Fry (1989) put it, the moral ideal of caring is unique to nursing and its moral commitment or covenant with society. It is that which distinguishes nursing ethics from medical, biomedical, traditionalist and rationalist ethics. It is the feminine

scholarship, systems and our society, when such are shaped by psyche, minds and bodies so influenced by war and by public professional knowledge and history informed by the masculine, the fight, the war and the non-caring?

What is there to say when even today we hide and deny that shaping? Can women and nurses, and nursing as a profession, with an ethic and ethos of caring, have any voice when we too have assembled as stones, circling around the troops or wagons holding terrible secrets? We have assembled as stones with only a small refrain, not even a chorus, and certainly no full voice as yet.

Do not despair. It is on occasions like these that we should exhume the stories of those stones of caring and reconsider the power of stones in the stream as stepping stones, helping us to create a map-in-the making of an alternate route.

So, from one century to another, ethical caring challenges for nursing and nurse scholars (both inside and outside the academic community of today and tomorrow) are the same as they were over 100 years ago. Similar challenges related to caring ethics continue to dominate as we enter the next century. For example, in 1852, Florence Nightingale asked the rhetorical question, which haunts us today as then, 'Why have women passion, intellect, moral activity—these three, and a place in society where not one of the three can be exercised?' (Nightingale 1979).

A hundred years or so later, even to this very moment (in 1997), scholars in nursing and related fields of education, philosophy, women's studies and so on, are still grappling with responses to Nightingale's question.

Almost eight decades after Nightingale's writing in 1859, Virginia Woolf's existential project *Three Guineas* (1938) asks a similar question on this topic:

If we encourage the daughters (and now sons) of educated men to enter the professions, shall we not be encouraging the very qualities we wish to prevent? [war, non-caring, violence].

... if we encourage (them) to enter the professions without making any conditions as to the

principle trying to be born in the work and world of nursing that is emerging in nursing and other disciplines at this point in our collective history and in medicine and nursing's modern traditions.

Studies have affirmed that nurses rely on a moral response of care and caring (attention to details of the patient's experiences; the principle of beneficence, relation, context, and so on), including highly valued responsiveness and sensitivity to the patient's wishes. This is in contrast with the physician's valuing of the scientific and distancing approaches to patient care and decision making (Peter & Gallop 1994, p. 47). Noddings (1989) indicated in her work on women and evil that an 'utter and absolute gap' (p. 126) exists between doctors and nurses; she repeats Doris Lessing's question: 'How did this extraordinary system grow up, where those who issue orders don't know what is really going on?' One problem Noddings (1989) acknowledges is that physicians do not participate in the extended intervals of direct caring that nurses see as the heart of their work. They do not have an equal opportunity to show their caring but, as she points out, they do not develop genuine attitudes of caring because they do not undertake the hands-on work that engenders such attitudes.

Touching is an example that Noddings uses. Touch is a central part of nursing but not of doctoring. She notes that touch is an act of valuing that exemplifies the unity in reciprocity of language, body, culture and nature and that communicates the complexity and diversity of nurses' values, their worth in different contexts and their identity (Noddings 1989, p. 126).

The nursing research on ethics and caring also converges with Gilligan's (1982) model of care, justice, moral development and gender-related work on caring ethics and the feminine, as developed by Noddings. In spite of this work, we know that caring and the woman's voice have largely been submerged in a culture of silence, overwhelmed by official declamation, by technical tasks, and by medical and scientific media formulations of both 'truth' and 'reality'.

An interesting turn is in what columnist Ellen Goodman calls 'revisionist medicine': the endless number of twists and turns in the plot of modern medicine and modern reality, distorting methods of all

way in which the professions are to be practised, shall we not be doing our best to stereotype the old tune, which human nature, like a gramophone whose needle has stuck, is now grinding out with such disastrous unanimity?

... shall we swear that the professions in the future shall be practiced so that they lead to a different song and a different conclusion ...?

(Woolf 1938, p. 59)

sorts to justify means. One month breast implants are safe, the next month unsafe; one day mastectomy is the only solution for breast cancer, the next biopsy; one day invasive surgery, another day 'non-invasive' radiation. While these changes are brought on by new research discoveries, all of this conveys a lack of any sense of professional moral community.

Such turns leave us breathless with respect to ethical challenges and the lack of caring in the academic, scientific, professional and public community. When, informed by nursing's core values, we enter into ethical caring challenges in academe and professional life, we call forth an existential project of acting on our caring ideals, which involves a rejection of what Maxine Greene calls 'the insufficient or the unendurable, a clarification, an imaging of a better state of things' (Greene 1988, p. 5). This is what Noddings (1989) called a 'yearning for the good'.

However, we are not enabled to reach out for conscious change if we are not able to 'name' the obstacles that stand in our way. Recently, nurse scholars, feminist writers, critical theorists, educators, existential philosophers and others have begun, like Nightingale and Woolf before us, to name the obstacles that stand in the way of liberating the human condition for freedom and caring.

As Maxine Greene reminds us, the point is not that there are never any excuses, but that, in classrooms as well as in the open world, accommodations come too easily. It is the case, as Sartre (1963) said, that there is an 'anguish' linked to action on one's caring, an anguish due to the recognition of one's own responsibility for what is happening (Greene 1988, p. 5).

As one of my professional nursing students, an experienced operating room nurse, said to me: 'Every day it takes courage, and I have to remind myself every day that "It is through courage to care that I get through the day in my system; it is *so* hard and I feel all alone".' The concept of moral courage comes into play here. As a pressing issue for the postmodern crisis of values presents itself, we awaken to it and name it.

Questions arise as to how we are to counter (in the name of caring) what Michel Foucault (1984) called 'power'—that which inheres in prevailing discourse and in knowledge itself (Greene 1988, p. 4). The language of contemporary schooling and of proposed reforms emphasizes something quite different from interpretative, critical, reflective thinking. Rather than being challenged to attend to the actualities of their lives as they are lived, students are urged to attend to what is 'given' in the outside world, whether in the form of 'high technology' or in the form of information. Educational reform often results in people learning more, having more content and more factual, empirical knowledge, rather than *being* more, the necessary ingredient for a caring community.

On the other hand, science scholars and historians are now mounting a many-sided attack on the central Western philosophical tradition of knowledge and science. It has been criticized as a futile exercise in linguistic game playing; a sustained but doomed effort to move beyond the elaborate fictions of its own creation (Tarnas 1993). The modern profession, with its models of knowledge and science, has been further condemned as being inherently alienating and oppressively hierarchical and competitive, leading to existential and cultural impoverishment and technocratic, non-caring domination of others and nature. It is not only self-deceptive, but war making and destructive. As Joseph Campbell (1972, p. 179) pointed out, the two greatest works of war in the West are the Iliad and the Old Testament. In some of this literature, the enemy is handled as though he were subhuman: not a 'thou' (to use Martin Buber's (1965) term), but a thing, an 'it' (Campbell 1972, p. 181). At many levels in our Western literature we have been bred on brutal war mythologies.

Richard Tarnas, in his remarkable book *The Passion of the Western Mind* (1993, p. 400), summarizes the plight and struggles of the 20th century, bringing forth the haunting refrains of Virginia Woolf and Florence Nightingale, which linger still:

Postmodern critical thought has encouraged a vigorous rejection of the entire western, intellectual 'canon', as long defined and privileged by a more or less exclusively male, white, European elite. Received truths concerning man, reason, civilization and progress are indicted as intellectually and morally bankrupt.

Under the cloak of western value, too many sins have been committed. Disenchanted eyes are not cast onto the west's long history of ruthless expansionism and exploitation ... its colonialism and imperialism, its slavery and genocide, its ... oppression of women, people of color, minorities, homosexuals, the working classes, the poor, its destruction of indigenous societies throughout the world, its arrogant insensitivity to other cultural traditions and values, its cruel abuse of other forms of life, its blind ravaging of virtually the entire planet ....

The contemporary academic world has increasingly concerned itself with the critical deconstruction of traditional assumptions, leading to a hermeneutics of suspicion. Postmodernism is deconstruction, decentering, disappearance, dissemination, demystification, discontinuity, difference, *dispersions and so on. It is an obsession with fragments or fractures.*   (Tarnas 1993, p. 401)

In spite of its contextual caring focus and intentionality for human sensitivity and moral community, nursing has in many ways decontextualized from itself and, in addition, has been 'decontextualized' from academia and the professional and public world of practice. Recent texts and hermeneutic studies in the nursing curriculum deconstruct this phenomenon, reflecting how the academic world has perpetuated the Western ethic of knowledge and science. For example, Hiraki's (1992, pp. 1–12) work, a critical hermeneutic study on 'tradition, rationality and power' in introductory nursing textbooks, revealed the kinds of 'professionalism' and normative structures of what constitutes authority and responsibility in nursing education, research, and practice.

Hiraki's study investigated the language used to describe, explain and interpret nursing in commonly used nursing textbooks. In spite of all historical and extant nursing philosophers, theorists and ethics scholars of the past few decades who have endorsed the caring ethical relationship and process, it seems that nursing is still defined by 'doing', by tradition, and by strict rationality and power, not by a human caring ethic or ethos.

In critiquing four of the most commonly used nursing textbooks, those fundamental texts which dictate what is legitimate knowledge, Hiraki found (1992, p. 2):

- the meaning of nursing practice in fundamental nursing textbooks is unquestionably determined by a rationality and language that strongly favors nursing as technical
- standardization (of nursing) is based on the assumption that nursing care can be translated into a scientific problem-solving process.

She found that this technical view of nursing was uncritically accepted by nurses in both practice and education. The assumption that caring can be translated into a technical, mechanistic, problem-solving strategy was unquestioned. The extreme objectification of particular forms of knowing, such as caring, perpetuates unethical caring practices and the status quo. Such strict rationalist thinking provides a guide for action, a theory that is not applicable to a world of values, a world of human relationship, ambiguities, meanings, cultural symbols and feeling. It separates factual knowledge from both values and human meanings.

In each instance, in all four textbooks, Hiraki found that the historical narrative about nursing acknowledged the primacy–authority of empirical, analytic traditions of science. Science was viewed as neutral, totally unbiased and value free. She points out: 'value-free metaphors decontextualized and limited nursing practice to a historical, objectified way of relating to the world' (Hiraki 1992, p. 2).

The domination of the science and technical metaphor in our knowledge, texts, practices and research methods eliminates the authenticity of human caring practices, the inner-life world and experiences of meaning. In the deconstructed nursing texts, even when considering humanistic communication of compassion, trust and other altruistic qualities, there was still reliance on objective behavior as the arbiter of a professional relationship.

All the texts conveyed a belief that a real scientific base for nursing with legitimate, rational forms of knowledge would be the solution to nursing's autonomy and professional development problems. Hiraki's work reminds us of Virginia Woolf's question: 'Should we encourage the daughters … to enter the professions without making any conditions as to the way in which the professions are to be practiced … ?' (Woolf 1938)

The concern with an ethic of caring in academe and practice parallels the ethics of caring in health care and society generally. In all aspects, we confer expertise and authority to technological and scientific knowledge while failing to recognize the other dimensions of human existence and life. We fail to realize that the system is wounded.

Moccia (1994) pointed out that when nurses in the 1960s sought out higher education as a means of escape from the patriarchal, oppressive and, in too many instances, abusive patterns of nursing in hospitals, they found that the supposed freedoms they would enjoy were illusory. Nurses found that higher education itself was (and still is) in turmoil. There was (and still is) an absence of an ethic or even a vision of caring.

As Moccia put it, we have not yet envisioned alternatives to the status quo in institutions of higher education, or in health care, nor have we attempted to design or redesign them. We are still lacking the awareness of a need to do things radically and fundamentally different. She framed the challenges for nursing educators and scholars: 'Where do our loyalties lie, and with whom do we wish to make alliance? And to whose good?' (Moccia 1994, pp. 472–474).

Moccia also cites Virginia Woolf with respect to our 'unreal loyalties', or perhaps our misplaced, distorted or deformed loyalties. In the past, she asserts, nursing's loyalties have been to its hospitals; most recently, they have been to programs or schools of nursing. At the same time, nursing has argued that its loyalty belongs to the patient or client and to its communities. Our past and recent history shows that nursing and academe have been distracted from these loyalties. What is called for at this point in our history—the point of transition between the modern loyalties to our systems—is to deconstruct, uncover, or expose the 'unreal loyalties' which keep us tied to modern institutions, rather than to the people we serve, to the students, clients, patients, communities and even to self.

As we deconstruct and expose the modern era, we see that the institutions that claim our loyalties are not health enterprises. They are not bad or evil or malevolent but they represent the masculine archetype as a dysfunctional paradigm for a postmodern awakening, an awakening to a realization that this worldview no longer works. The modern systems no longer care for our communities and our people; they no longer provide visions of caring, health and healing; they no longer nourish the intellect, spirit or soul of the participants (Moccia 1994, p. 473). Moccia reminds us of Audre Lorde's words that 'the Master's tools will never dismantle the master's house'.

At this point in nursing's evolution into the postmodern and beyond, we now resist unreal loyalties and masculine archetype principles as the answer to our ethical, scientific and professional practice challenges. Our loyalties at this point need to be with healing ourselves and our wounded systems. Leaving the masculine energy domination and unreal loyalties to the modern morality of the 20th century, it is time for nursing to work toward instituting its caring morality, to work on its own healing from inside out: from personal to system; from private spaces of pain to a transformation of the public world of education, science and practice (Moccia 1994, pp. 472–474).

7

Reconstructing nursing

....

We see other alternatives when a new light falls on our pain and
suffering and it then becomes unbearable. (adapted from Sartre, 1963)

Nursing redefining itself

At some deep level in human history, with
primordial truths of existence, there is a
knowing and experiencing with which we
long to reconnect, seeking the point of intersection of time with the timeless (Plate 3).

> Seeking the point of intersection:
> the plane that connects heaven
> and earth,
> time and timeless, Yin and Yang.

The classic Chinese Taoists described the concept that all of life is com-
prised of, and has been set in motion by, the constant interplay of two vital
energies: 'the principles of the passive Yin (everything female) and the
active Yang (everything male). In this cosmology, Yin and Yang together
give rise to everything in the world—"the ten thousand things"' (Shepherd
1993, p. 8).

As Shepherd explains, in the Yin–Yang system no part has a life of its
own, but each exists in complementary interaction with the other. Yin and
Yang mutually help each other; together they constitute equilibrium and
harmony. Though opposites, they need not be in opposition or antagonism, as often experienced in the male/female discourse of the present era.

Though different, they supplement, nourish and complete each other. They are the two vital energies giving rise to everything in the world, with everything acting as a continuous dance and movement between them, without a beginning and without end.

Nursing and medicine can represent an archetypal balance in health care; there is no need therefore for a hierarchy of superior or inferior qualities, knowledge and practices. Nursing and medicine become the different components required for harmonious treatment, curing and healing processes; they both become necessary parts of the whole. Society, in turn, becomes the benefactor and recipient: it gets the best that medicine and nursing together offer as a whole system, not as a duality where both compete for the same Yang energy, sacrificing one for the other.

This way of thinking does not deny the fact that nursing, as feminine energy, or Yin, contains a spot of masculine medicine. Likewise, within Yang medicine there is a dot of nursing, the Yin energy. The movement of both is like a wave; it represents the continuity of the life force and the search for wholeness, completion and harmony. It is probably helpful therefore to consider the Yang–Yin dimensions not as a duality but as a dance of differences, adding energy and wholeness to life and life processes (see Table 7.1).

The universality of the Yin and Yang principles lies dormant in the collective consciousness of all people and all civilizations. It symbolizes the creative yet oppressive tension that has existed throughout the rise of modern medicine and modern nursing. Ashley's (1976) early feminist critique of nursing's history illustrated how Yang the medical curing system has been, at the expense of nursing, symbolized by the caring Yin. Her account highlighted how many men in medicine, health care and hospital administration have kept nurses powerless, and have inhibited the growth of nursing as a caring profession.

Table 7.1 Yang and Yin, the universal masculine and feminine principles (From 'Lifting the Veil' by Linda Jean Shepherd © 1993, reprinted by arrangement with Shambhala Publications, Inc., Boston, and 'Between Heaven and Earth' by Harriet Beinfield and Efren Korngold © 1991, reprinted by permission of Ballantine Books, a division of Random House, Inc., New York.)

Yang	Yin
Masculine principle	Feminine principle
Right	Left
Revealed, expanding	Hidden, contracting
Primal power	Yielding, substantive
Active, dynamic	Receptive, passive
Thinking, responsive, expressive	Feelings, thoughts
Logos, the objective, factual, logical	Eros, the principle of relatedness
Knowledge for the sake of knowledge	Application of knowledge, co-creation of knowledge
Analytic	Comprehensive
Disciplinary	Non-disciplinary
Order	Chaos, pattern
Accomplishment, efficiency	Pleasure, enjoyment
Experiment, adventure	Security, familiarity, openness
Competition	Sense of community
Head, intelligence	Soul, body
Sense information	Intuition
Tangible, rational, objective	Intangible, subjective, intersubjective
Concentration, determination	Relaxation, fluidity
Pursuit, construction	Receptivity, maintenance
Hard	Soft
Fire, air	Earth, water
Dry	Moist
Light, day	Dark, night
Sun	Moon
Hot	Cold
Summer	Winter
Positive	Negative
Vertical	Horizontal
Meat	Vegetables
(Heaven)	(Earth)

While American hospitals were established by men to offer nursing care, the care was actually provided by women/nurses who worked essentially as indentured servants, until very recent times. The male physicians and hospital administrators were preoccupied with control over others, profits and (male) privileges. The female nurses (and growing numbers of male nurses) were committed to service, to health education and to the welfare of students and patients: to the human caring processes. These nursing functions eventually were discouraged by medical men and the systems of cure, adding to nursing's current demise. This vast, largely unacknowledged, cultural value difference between men in medicine and women in nursing has accelerated and polarized some of the contemporary crises in both fields. This time of transition is a time to harmonize the imbalance between the Yin and Yang, the conflicsts of medical and nursing values, and to maximize the point where they intersect, thus creating a new whole.

In 1944, Anne Morrow Lindburgh apprehended the remarkable, time-less intersection of differences between years and time, something she referred to as a realization of an intersection between two planes of existence. She remarked that usually we move on one plane of existence, the physical, Yang, outer world, but occasionally, in moments of elation, danger, deep joy, or during transitions, crises and vulnerable moments in our life or our plane of existence, whether personal or professional, we find ourselves transferred to the (Yin) plane of the uncommon, providing us with a sense of cosmic perspective.

This postmodern era is an era between cosmologies, an era in-between a sense of the profane and the divine; the obscene and the sacred. Perhaps we are again in search of that plane between this time and the timeless past which will reconnect us with the deep, archetypal level of human existence and contribute to the creation of a new future. Perhaps that is what the new millennium will bring: a future that no longer has a need to rank along the patriarchal, masculine/feminine value scale.

Maybe, for the next turn in our history, we can find the intersection between the two planes of existence, between the timeless, sacred, archetypal societies and cosmologies which have represented peace and life-generating forces, and have flourished without war and without hierarchy. This time in history knows its need for reordering its imbalance between the secular and the sacred (Fig. 7.1). In this time of intersection we can

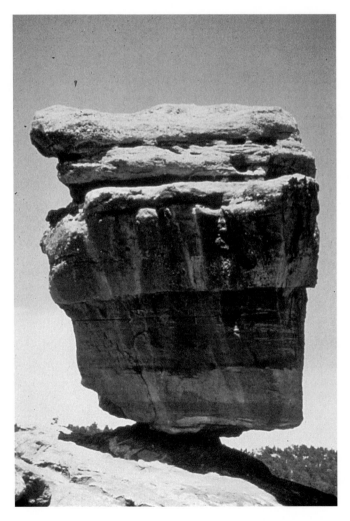

Figure 7.1 At this time in history we need to find a balance between the secular and the sacred. (Photograph by Dr Chantal Cara. Reproduced with permission.)

no longer frame diversity as inferiority or superiority; neither can half of humanity be ranked superior to the other.

As in the prehistoric cosmology, perhaps once again we can find the point in this time that intersects with the timeless approaches that link and connect, rather than rank and separate; that create partnerships, rather than domination; that seek non-linear, possibly invisible, creative, harmonizing forces and possibilities, rather than force the ever-visible, tangible, linear sameness and search for, manipulate and control perpetual predictabilities.

Intersections between world and time

Today, many people are trying to reach the point which intersects and connects with deeper meanings and truths created in the path of our time. We see a search for the spirit and the spiritual at every turn: if not angels, then at least shamans. We need only visit a bookstore to see the quest for the point of intersection with the timeless. It is all laid out before us: the 'Search for the beloved', the 'Care of the soul', 'Recovering the soul', 'In search of the soul', 'God and the new physics', 'Fire in the soul'; 'Code for the soul', and so on. This time is being propelled to a point that we do not yet know, nor can we apprehend where it may take us, but something is 'going on'. Indeed, as the theologian and geologist Thomas Berry suggested, human(s) may now be defined as the latest expression of the cosmic–earth process, as that being in whom the process becomes conscious of itself.

What is 'going on', it seems to me, takes us back to the deep archetypal meaning of life's force and energy for creation and survival. This is where woman and nurse stand as a timeless, yet dynamic, value-laden archetype (see Glossary of definitions, p. 285) in the midst of a search for that point of intersection between time and the timeless (Plate 1). This search aims to embrace the near and far in the same instant and to seize the tangible, manifestly real essence and the divine, against the backdrop of the surreal and the virtually real. It aims to synthesize the concrete with the abstract, the factual with the spiritual and the superficial with the sacred.

Kech (1995) described 'what is going on', and this deep-value intersection point, from the standpoint of humankind 'growing up', moving from Epoch I, through Epoch II and entering into Epoch III. Each historical epoch has contributed to humankind's evolution and further development in the universe.

Kech's Epoch I is equated with the birth and childhood of humanity: the physical plane development. According to his views and deep-value trend analysis, Epoch I was reached between 50 000 and 100 000 years ago, when we realized we were part of a larger world and subject to forces beyond ourselves.

Epoch II, through which we are currently living at this point in our history, commenced about 10 000 years ago, when we matured into our 'collective adolescence'. The focus has been on ego and mental development and the value system has essentially been masculine, with the heavy Yang energy of the patriarchy and all that has generated, for better and for worse.

The convergence for the 'intersection of time with the timeless' that Lindberg (1944) wrote about is manifesting itself as we leave the 20th century and enter into Epoch III. This epoch is symbolized by the 'coming of age of humanity' into its adulthood. It is this epoch which brings with it the transformation of the human psyche as the deep soul energies (of the Yin) call us forth to move toward spiritual maturation. It is in this epoch that we seek wholeness in body, mind and spirit, and oneness with the universe. Kech goes so far as to indicate that if we do not move forward for this next phase of maturity for humanity, we actually may abort our human evolutionary journey. He also cautions that a transitional time such as this is 'our collective "dark night of the soul"' (Kech 1995, p. 6). It is a dark night because what we have known within the so-called 'modern' era is dying. What was formerly our daylight is no longer, within the post-modern dismantling and awakening that is occurring. He emphasizes that this time of transition and transformation is dark for the soul because it involves the soul and the archetypal, deep-value aspects of our life. It involves the soul because it is about spiritual development.

Kech makes the transformative metamorphosis connection with the soul emerging. He reminds us that the Greek word for 'soul' is the same as the word used for 'butterfly'. The butterfly (Yin, creative birthing) energy is also what is contained within the chrysalis, which allows us to meta-morphose ourselves from sickness into health as a civilization and an evolved humankind.

Extant nursing discourse is being redefined within Epoch III. The deep archetypal value shift in our philosophies, theories and practices contains emerging themes as the context and processes for health. These themes include the unity of mind, body and spirit, inner human potential and inner healing processes, healing environments, expanding consciousness, the human–environment–nature–universe field and energy source, spiritu-ality and soul care. These are all Epoch III, Yin themes and stand in con-trast to conventional, Yang, Epoch II medical themes. These themes come from a different source. They border on the sacred and are indeed linked with the sacred. They connect the feminine principle with the sacred universe, unfolding.

> *The soul is often imagined to be feminine. All those qualities thought of as soulful, a dreaminess or artistic sensibility, are supposed to come more naturally to women. Ephemeral, half-seen, half-present, nearly ghostly, with only the vaguest relation to the practical world of physical law, the soul appears to us as lost. The hero, with his more masculine virtues, must go in search of her. But there is another, older story of the soul. In this story she is firmly planted on the earth. She is incarnate and visible everywhere. Neither is she faint of heart, nor fading in her resolve. It is she, in fact, who goes bravely in search of desire.* (Griffin 1992, p. 132).

In the most pronounced directions that go beyond the postmodern 'post–postmodern' developments in nursing and other areas, there is an attempt to recover the deep, hidden, archetypal sacred, which is the feminine. This is not just about male and female, but is about a universal experience. It is a universal human capacity and a basic human need.

When this deep, archetypal, sacred, human need is unfulfilled, we become wounded and ill, as a people, a society, a culture, a world and a planet. We are all part of and we all belong to this process and this timeless search for access to the sacred.

Remen (1994) reminds us that recovery of the sacred is not about 'something more'; it is not about adding on to yourself, nor fixing yourself. The sacred is not acquired; it is remembered. It is about retrieving that which we have hidden from ourselves, individually and collectively.

The loss of the sacred came with the loss of respect for the feminine archetypal energy and the feminine life-giving connecting principles. The feminine is 'the doorway, the royal road to the sacred' (Remen 1994, p. 124). Without the feminine, we are cut off from the very process that heals.

As nursing redefines itself for this emerging post–postmodern millennium, it is its feminine principle that it brings as access to the sacred, as the secret of healing. Without nursing healing its own wounds and recovering its own energy source, it ceases to exist. Just as medicine will cease to exist without restoring the sacred within its practices.

The point of intersection proposed in this book, which goes beyond the postmodern deconstructions, attempts to find, connect and reconstruct the two planes of the deep archetypal intersection of the masculine and femi-nine principles. While the feminine may be historically imaged as weak and retiring, in this story the nurse is firmly planted on the earth, becoming incarnate and visible, holding up the light and the metaphorical mirror to the soul; 'connecting the earth plane with the heavenly, the divine'. Neither is she faint of heart, nor fading in her resolve. It is she who goes bravely in search of how things might be, rather than accepting what is.

There are, however, no experts in this matter. It is a philosophy, a way of seeing and a way of experiencing, participating and manifesting what already is, which we all have access to. This process of honoring and revaluing the feminine principle is what Mary Catherine Bateson (1990) called 'practiced improvisation'; it is part of what nursing is and what composing a life is. For me, it is exposing *and* composing a life and a profession for the 21st century.

The other option is to ignore the attempt to *see* anything different or differently; to ignore the desire to *be* anything different or differently; to refuse to ask 'What ails thee?' and seek to restore it:

> *... we didn't even inquire, didn't even see how the rest was going on ... all these things were happening and we didn't see them.* (Briggs & Peat 1991, p. 203)

To go in search of the older story of the soul, into the sea of our (un)consciousness, while we uncover the one-sidedness of the archetypal imbalance, we rediscover and remember those parts which enhance the whole. The other side emerges into a new profession, informed by nursing's feminine principles, but workable and needed for health and all health practitioners (Newman et al 1991). For example, as the ancient archetypal feminine principles, symbolized by nursing, begin to manifest into a mature paradigm, we see the following structure emerge:

- The result: nursing, both manifesting and simultaneously transcending its caring–healing paradigm.
- The paradox: nursing is no longer nursing, as we have known it within the modern era; it has become something else, more nursing, not less.

These old/new, modern/postmodern, nursing/medicine aspects embrace, encompass and invite participation in the sacred feminine principles as the philosophical and moral foundation for professional models of caring–healing practices which include:

- Honoring deeper, subjective meanings and feelings about life, living, the natural inner processes and choices.
- Considering the relational, intuitive and receptive rather than the separatist and disconnected ways of knowing and being; honoring art, beauty and aesthetics together with science and technology.
- Living, researching and practicing from a call motivated by love: a love of life, humans, nature and all living things.
- Discovering ourselves through the forms of inquiry rather than a desire to control or 'know' an isolated event which stands outside ourselves.
- Incorporating intersubjectivity, feelings, unknowns, transcendence, mystery and even chaos into our life, work and play.
- Seeking nurturing, cooperation, multiplicity, relatedness and harmony in our relations with self, others, nature and the planet (Plate 2).
- Following an inner and outer vision of wholeness and healing.

The modern Western medicine lens became nurses' and nursing's lens for seeing their reality and phenomena. When we stop observing our glasses, or the color or shape of our lens, we forget we are wearing them. That doesn't mean, however, that they are not affecting us. Indeed, our lens refracts the world and lights up, diffuses and covers over our reality in ways that alter our view of person, man, woman, nature, health, illness, caring, curing, healing and our systems and institutions. Our glasses define our sense of right and wrong, that which we consider humane and scientific in our practices and whether and how we consider a higher/deeper divinity.

The modern lens of nursing, medicine, Western science and the Western world refracted out the feminine principle from nursing and humankind. Some say the repression of the feminine in our world is a measure of pathology; a pathology of society that inhibits our further evolution and generativity.

Both we and our modern systems have been wounded at all turns. Simultaneously, the modern Western cosmology lost its center, hence the postmodern condition of free-floating angst. A culture and medical system without a center is a culture and medical system in crisis, wounded. The wounds of this juncture are universal wounds in that we have all become wounded in the same way.

Joseph Campbell (1972) names our woundedness: because we have cut ourselves off from our myths, meanings and symbols, we have lost the sacred and the soul. The sacred and the soul are universal, part of the human condition. Remembering and thus recovering the sacred feminine archetype of nursing is remembering something we have forgotten and, at times, even hidden from ourselves. Recovering and remembering nursing qua nursing now requires us to remove the modern lens of nursing and medicine. To recover nursing within the postmodern era and beyond we have to look deeply into our own Venus's mirror for the sacred feminine. In looking into a different mirror or through a different lens, we must throw away the old glasses. They no longer work or serve as a lens through which to see the changing world. We must release our mindset and belief system, even our cherished values. The remembering of the sacred now requires some forgetting of the modern.

This remembering is an ethical and scientific challenge for nursing. The postmodern does not define it for us; it only reminds us that there has been a culture-wide forgetting and devaluing of what we have forgotten. The sacred feminine archetype principle has been used across time as a road to the sacred. Without it we cut ourselves off from our life source.

In considering nursing within an emerging cosmology for the 21st century and the next age in humankind, the model of postmodern nursing captures an evolving, covolving universe that once again honors the sacred feminine. Whether this honoring comes from nursing as exemplar, or from medicine, other health professions, or the public, it seeks to go beyond what is and projects what might be.

Changing the lens: a new looking glass

Will we carry reductionism on toward the ultimate dream (and perhaps ultimate deception) ... or will we enter the turbulent mirror (Venus') embracing our limitations (destructive direction) and acknowledging our dependence (on creative, life-giving forces)?   (Briggs & Peat 1990, p. 202)

The turbulent mirror is Venus's mirror. It serves as a looking glass into the modern–postmodern crisis in science and society. It also serves as an image through which to view the ontological transition which is already transforming our being for the next era in human history.

Collectively and symbolically, nursing serves as a psychic archetype which can be a mirror for society. It stands as a looking glass through which to understand the complexities and paradoxes of the ontological shift occurring within the postmodern world of medicine, nursing and the Western world. Nursing's emergence at a deeper archetypal level is a metaphor that helps us see into the glass 'darkly', while recognizing the emerging caring–healing cosmology that is remembering the sacred feminine.

Caring is both old and new. As something old it is tradition, literally something that has been handed on in the oral tradition of women (and enlightened men) as folklore through time: the timeless. As something new, it is thinking in ways that mix the tradition and past wisdoms with a new awakening of caring knowledge and moral ideals and practices to counter the social crises of the modern era. With the new lens for seeing, we seek the point of intersection between the time and the timeless, the heaven and the earth, the masculine and feminine spirit of our ground of being (Plate 3).

The paradox and illusions of reality are being mirrored from the modern lens to the postmodern. Paradoxically, nursing as metaphor and symbol mirrors the wounds of the modern Western medical system. It now needs to fully embrace its own wounds in order to heal itself. This is the time to move from a place of unconsciousness (of its vital energy), away from its self-consciousness to another place of owning its own inner strength.

This new place heals by deconstructing and decentering the past oppression and unconsciousness. This new/old place awakens nursing and women/men to an evolved consciousness whereby it remembers itself, connects with, claims and mirrors its deepest power outwardly. Nursing then learns to hold its sacred mirror light to the world.

Caring–healing model

The next section of this book lays out the paradigm shift and the emerging caring–healing model that reflects and mirrors the highest/deepest actualization of nursing qua nursing, within the sacred feminine archetype. The model simultaneously and paradoxically transcends. Nursing, redefined with the sacred feminine, becomes a model for 21st century nursing and medicine and perhaps for all health care providers.

Venus's mirror images nursing's prophecy and legacy and presents itself as a paradigm case—the holder of the mirror of the ancient Yin—for the emerging Epoch III era of human history. Nursing's legacy offers a voice for the caring–healing needed for this time between worlds. Modern humankind either rediscovers its own soul or destroys itself and the planet Earth as we have known it.

Nursing has a covenant with itself and humankind which is now being rebirthed, for now and the next 100 years of evolving humankind. If it is not able to fulfill that convenant, it may not survive. It either matures into its own sacred healing practices, or remains in a technical, dependent position within the patriarchal system of medicine.

It is an interesting and provocative choice that we are called to make at this crossroads in our history, during this time of transition between worlds and time. Caring in nursing, as archetype, invites an awakening of a long-lost tradition: that of rediscovering new life and vitality for nurses and others who want to enter into this discovery and move with the release of new energy into professional life practices. It is for nurses who want to incorporate this new release and vitality into nursing's disciplinary development, who want to use social action and caring, to flow into and awaken others, to offer nursing's caring–healing consciousness as a creative outlet for the whole.

This caring–healing model is rooted in Nightingale and in caring theory; it draws upon a converging of nursing's contemporary, emerging paradigm. It is both theoretical and beyond theory. It is located within the postmodern discourse, but also goes beyond that toward reconstructing the dormant margin that has been always, already, inscribed in the history of women. The reconstructed nursing model is ironically beyond nursing. It now serves as a model for the whole. The transition from modern to postmodern is more than a subtle shift; it is transformative. It requires a new pair of glasses—a new lens to see both old and new phenomena in different ways.

So, at this point, we go beyond modern and postmodern, beyond deconstructing, even beyond nursing. In shifting toward Epoch III and the new millennium, we consider the transformative model for postmodern nursing and beyond, now located within a new sacred feminine cosmology that has relevance to all health professionals and humankind.

Transpersonal nursing as ontological *artist*

8

Beyond postmodern nursing —into the next millenium

A more complete study of the movements of the world will oblige us, little by little, to turn it upside down ...   (Teilhard de Chardin 1959, p. 43)

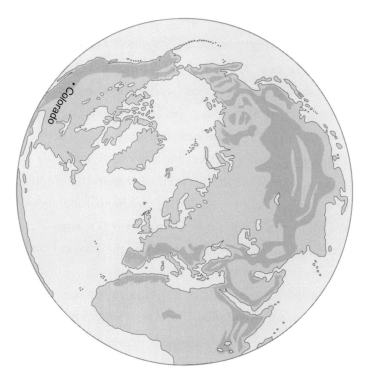

Figure 8.1 Postmodern/transpersonal nursing requires a new worldview, in which the world may be turned 'upside down', as each is challenged to relocate the self within a new world order.

If we were to take seriously the disclosure of an ontological and epistemological bias in Western science ... (there are) ... a whole set of archetypal realities waiting to be discovered, at the highest reaches of the human consciousness, by all people.

(Harman 1991, p. 8, Rossner 1989)

A caring–healing cosmology and ontological shift

The art and science of human caring and healing can be considered in some ways *autopoietic*; that is, it has been and is a discipline that is making itself. Perhaps it is true that the roots of caring science and service come from nursing, but now, as caring evolves into a more distinct focus in relation to its importance for inner healing and health outcomes for self-caring and self-recovery, something new presents itself.

This 'something new' is placing nursing's conventional, marginalized theories, philosophies and practices within the cosmology of emerging 21st century thinking. This new cosmology is based on a foundational shift at the ontological level. This new, emerging, postmodern-and-beyond discipline of nursing now intersects much more closely with philosophy, art and humanities, feminist studies, ethics and moral development theory, creating new views of science (including psychoneuroimmunology (PNI) and the quantum theory of physics) and deep, archetypal connections between the physical and spiritual, between the physical and the non-physical, and between the physical and metaphysical. All of this allows nursing to take another giant step or leap toward remaking and redefining itself, thus giving it room and possibilities it never had before.

This new space for nursing to redefine itself is possible, whether one still locates nursing within the passing modern paradigm, or moves forward within the postmodern turn. As the momentum accelerates for nursing science and practice, nursing suddenly finds itself, ironically, *beyond nursing*, while simultaneously being fully grounded in its roots. As nursing's models and practices of caring–healing continue to be clarified and advanced, and continue to be more consistent with its theories, philosophies and values, then nursing becomes a more distinct health–caring–healing profession. As this occurs, nursing's practices and professional education and research automatically converge with other practitioners and health professions, within those 'indeterminate zones' of caring and healing.

This section seeks to clarify what the new evolved paradigm is becoming —this paradigm that is ironically nursing and yet beyond nursing. The emerging new paradigm (see Table 8.1) represents the cosmological and ontological shift that is occurring as we take leave of one century and one millennium and enter another. As we do so, 'what is probably needed … is a qualitatively new theory, … to begin with what (we) have in common—undivided wholeness' (Bohm 1988).

Reconstructing for postmodern nursing and caring

Reconstruction of the so-called 'master narrative' of modern medicine and nursing is an attempt to locate and disclose nursing's caring–healing text and nursing's sacred feminine archetype from the margin. It is an attempt to reverse the resident hierarchy of medical control for caring and healing, to pry loose nursing qua nursing's paradigm in order to reconstitute what has already existed

Deconstructing the modern

As we continue peering into the abyss of the past, we can see its colour changing.   *(Teilhard de Chardin 1959, p. 74)*

Deconstructing can be defined as the attempt 'to locate the promising marginal text, to disclose the undecidable moment, to pry loose … to reverse the resident hierarchy, only to displace it; to dismantle in order to reconstitute what is always already inscribed' (Derrida 1976, in: Sarup 1988, p. 56). Within nursing, it is to go beyond 'modern' technology and masculine archetype medicine; it is to critique the human subject, the separatist ontology and morality that constitutes the professional–political–scientific–clinical hierarchy of the current system.   *(Watson 1995)*

Table 8.1 Nursing's transformative caring–healing paradigm

Modern	Postmodern/beyond
Cosmology: man/human-centered/ deterministic	Unitary consciousness, co-evolving; connectedness of all
Masculine warrior archetype	Sacred feminine archetype harmonizing Yin with Yang
Separatist ontology	Relational ontology
Physical/material phenomena	Non-physical/metaphysical; a new integration
Separateness science	Wholeness science
Technological competencies	Ontological competencies
Medical procedures, tasks, skills	Advanced caring–healing modalities: postmodern
Morality/value-hard science	Caring as ethic and moral foundation
Consciousness fixed, localized	Unitary consciousness; consciousness as energy
Caring means curing	Caring consciousness primary
Human: mindbodyspirit split	Mindbodyspirit oneness; human interconnected with nature, life processes
Person as machine: body physical	Embodied spirit; self-transcendence; soul, sacred
Time–space closed/absolute/fixed	Relativity of time–space, past–present–future
Reality: science, material world	Metaphor: art–artistry co-created; creative
Human–environment: control, separate	Person–nature–universe, oneness-interconnected
Health–illness: disease, external	Health as consciousness; human–environmental energy field
Health care institutions: modern technology, sterile, 'institutional'	Postmodern systems become archetypal dwelling: mind–body soul; microcosm for caring-healing needs
Dominant metaphor: science, technology, machine	Art, artistry, emergence of beauty, harmony, search for wholeness
Blade	Chalice–Blade unity
Yang	Yin–Yang balance
Production	Creation
Isolated, independent doing	Being-in-relation
Medicalizing of health and human experiences	Spiritualizing of health, inner healing

'as the promise, on the margin' of the medical–treatment center. It is to reconstruct a transformative paradigm of caring–healing praxis.

Redefining nursing from modern to postmodern translates caring values into an ontology of relation—a dramatic transformative cosmology and shift from the modern nursing paradigm. Modern nursing resides within a separatist ontology, consistent with Western science, which separates person from nature, and being from knowing and doing.

In this postmodern model of human caring, healing and wholeness become the starting points, the midpoints and the open endings for the ongoing, evolving and unfolding of the human condition. The post-modern opens to new ways of being human, of being-in-relation, in multi-dimensions and planes of existence in the universe.

One of the constraints of the postmodern era is that life continues to be free-floating and nebulous. As a result there is often a silence with respect to values and moral components. Values and texts have been deconstructed to an extreme, leaving humans empty and anxious in the ambiguity of relevance. However, in keeping with the deconstructing/reconstructing process within the postmodern, the reconstructing discloses caring as a moral ideal with the conscious intent to remember the sacred feminine and to preserve wholeness, potentiate healing and preserve dignity, integrity, and life-generating processes at the levels of human, nature and universe.

In positing postmodern nursing/beyond nursing as archetype, caring is an explicit global ontology of relation, rather than separation. It refers to a special way of being-in-relation as a moral starting point for caring for self, for higher/deeper self, other(s), nature and other living things on the planet Earth and in the broader universe. It calls forth a commitment to caring and an intentionality of a caring consciousness for the worlds of nursing and medicine, and also for the planet. It is located within a cosmology of oneness of consciousness, a consciousness of unity of mindbodyspirit and nature, what Bohm called 'unbroken wholeness' in the universe (Bohm 1988). This model is about the life-generating creative processes of life's energy forces, associated with Yin and with the sacred feminine archetype, as the ground of both nursing's being and that of beyond nursing. Nursing's evolving postmodern/beyond-nursing paradigm becomes an archetype for a transformed system.

Paradigms, possibilities, eras and evolutions

The nursing science literature has identified at least three paradigms that have affected nursing's progress and maturity as a discipline (Fawcett 1993, Newman 1992, Parses 1981):

- particulate–deterministic (Paradigm I)
- integrative–interactive (Paradigm II)
- unitary–transformative (Paradigm III).

The modern medical paradigms have also been categorized into three eras: Era I, Era II and Era III (Dossey 1991). These three eras of medical science and treatment models correspond to the three paradigms identified within the discipline of nursing.

Era I was associated with mechanism and materialism and with 'physical medicine'. It emphasized the body and the disease as functions of an objective world. Our bodies and their state became the focus for medical treatment and cure, from the outside in. This era considered people as 'bodies' for modern medical and nursing science.

This approach has dominated modern medicine and nursing practices and mindsets during the 20th century (Fig. 8.2). Nursing within Era I focused on material medicine and nursing; the fixation in this era became the functional tasks, skills and 'doing' role of nursing, which still continues

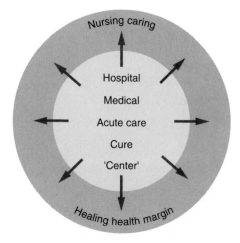

Figure 8.2 What is modern medicine/nursing?

throughout the United States and the Westernized world. Era I compares with the particulate–deterministic, Paradigm I era of nursing's evolution.

Era II medicine evolved into mind–body medicine (Epstein 1996), more properly meaning 'brain–body medicine', according to Dossey (1991), emphasizing the location of the mind in the brain. This era parallels the integrative–interactive Paradigm II period of nursing. In this era, from the mid 20th century onward, medical science, and consequently nursing education, science and practice, began to consider perceptions, emotions, attitudes and 'psychosomatic' perspectives in treatment and care practices.

The Era II/Paradigm II emergence in medicine/nursing parallels the rise of a 'patient-centered', psychosocial and emotional-needs focus in nursing education and, to a lesser extent, in nursing practice. This was the period of the 1960s onward, when psychiatric nursing and mental health concepts were integrated throughout nursing curricula, and practitioners experimented with team nursing. In nursing research, the 1970s and 1980s generated a critique of nursing research, knowledge and existing epistemology, a critique and deconstruction which still continues.

During the latter part of Era II/Paradigm II, there was a rapid increase in doctoral programs in nursing and a dramatic rise in the use of qualitative methods in research. There was increased attention in nursing research within a human science paradigm, and in practices related to patient-centered approaches, subjective experiences of pain, relaxation therapies, visualization, self-care and self-regulation, including patient-directed care. This fostered some of the early therapeutic touch and psychoneuro-immunology research, together with clinical intervention, communication, caring and outcome-based research, nursing and system redesign projects, and so on. Clinical practices focused on primary nursing and other models of comprehensive care, including nursing-managed centers.

The latter part of Era II/Paradigm II saw a rise in caring literature within nursing, and terms such as 'healing', 'spiritual' and even 'sacred', 'transcendent', 'energy' and 'consciousness' began to surface more frequently in the nursing literature. The same was true in related fields of practice, such as massage therapy, acupuncture and homeopathy, and the discipline of 'alternative medicine' was acknowledged more openly.

But Era II/Paradigm II mind–body concepts and practices in education, practice or research were never fully integrated into the modern framework of either medicine or nursing. Instead, they remained on the margin of Era I/Paradigm I, the dominant center despite the emergence of new knowledge and insights. There was certainly no mainstream effort to transform practice and education along mind–body medicine and nursing lines, although there was a great deal of rhetoric about the importance of Era II/Paradigm II thinking.

The attention given to complementary and alternative medicine during the late 1980s to the mid to late 1990s, along with the establishment of the National Institutes of Health Office of Complementary–Alternative Medicine (NIH-OCAM) in the USA and similar bodies elsewhere, became outward manifestations of a change in the mindset of the public and some practitioners. This awakening, however, remained tangential to what was still mainstream Era I/Paradigm I science and medical practices, even though those established practices were no longer working for the public or for the systems involved.

The exception was in nursing science. In the 1980s, human science models and research methods became more the norm, at least in some academic settings. But, while the shift continues to be in the direction of human science models for nursing research, these are still not considered to be representative of mainstream nursing science, even in the late 1990s.

Can nursing become something beyond what it has been during the Era I and Era II periods? Will Era III/Paradigm III nursing become something that is grounded in the premodern, spiritual traditions of Nightingale, yet will be something different for the future? There are signs that this will happen, and this book makes a case for that very position, but the answer is as yet unknown.

Nursing, at its deep archetypal level, and through the voices of its leaders across time, has always ascribed to a view of nursing that goes beyond Era I and Era II thinking. Nursing has held positions that have honored individuals with more than body-physical care and that have required more than the undertaking of a set of functional prescribed tasks, skills related to medical treatment protocols and cure-related activities. Nursing has always resisted stereotypes that define and represent nursing as 'doing'. Yet at the end of the 20th century, nursing still has to face some of the same struggles faced by Nightingale at the end of the 19th century (Newman et al 1991).

During the latter half of the 20th century, the 'redesign' and 're-engineering' mentality for health care reform has actually amounted to attempts to repair, fix or refinance an already broken model. The post-modern deconstruction of the conventional model and its basic masculine-principled ideologies has left medicine reeling from the shock of public and policy dismantling of the status quo. As a system, or society, we are trying to recover or repair the demise of medicine and nursing as they were organized within the industrial, material framework. This has led to a deeper level of reconstructing, thus allowing the emergence of a transformative model of caring and healing.

Even if nursing and medicine, as systems or as individual practitioners, are not ready to shift to a deeper Era III/Paradigm III transformation, and choose to fluctuate within the postmodern space, they can still change the lens they are using to engage in their work, and make a difference. They can learn to make an ontological shift in their way of being in relation to themselves and those they serve; they can choose to 'see' the sacred nature of the everyday. The really significant changes, however, come from a different way of seeing the world itself and of seeing how that opens up a new paradigm thinking which is truly transformative and different from what has come before.

The postmodern/transpersonal caring–healing Era III/Paradigm III

This reconstructed postmodern and beyond nursing (or medicine) model is emerging as the *transpersonal caring–healing Era III/Paradigm III*. The major assumptions of this are as follows:

- Caring is based on an ontology and ethic of relationship and connectedness, and of relationship and consciousness.
- Caring consciousness, in-relation, becomes primary.
- Caring can be most effectively demonstrated and practiced interpersonally and transpersonally.
- Caring consists of 'caritas' consciousness, values and motives. It is guided by carative components (see Watson 1995, 1988b, and Table 8.1, p. 96, for an overview of 'carative factors').

- A caring relationship and a caring environment attend to 'soul care': the spiritual growth of both the one-caring and the one-being-cared-for.

- A caring relationship and a caring environment preserve human dignity, wholeness and integrity; they offer an authentic presencing and choice.

- Caring promotes self-growth, self-knowledge, self-control and self-healing processes and possibilities.

- Caring accepts and holds safe space (sacred space) for people to seek their own wholeness of being and becoming, not only now but in the future, evolving toward wholeness, greater complexity and connectedness with the deep self, the soul and the higher self.

- Each caring act seeks to hold an intentional consciousness of caring. This energetic, focused consciousness of caring and authentic presencing has the potential to change the 'field of caring', thereby potentiating healing and wholeness.

- Caring, as ontology and consciousness, calls for ontological authenticity and advanced ontological competencies and skills. These, in turn, can be translated into professional ontologically based caring–healing modalities.

- The practice of transpersonal caring–healing requires an expanding epistemology and transformative science and art model for further advancement. This practice integrates all ways of knowing. The art and science of a postmodern model of transpersonal caring–healing is complementary to the science of medical curing, modern nursing and medical practices.

Some of the assumptions relating to a transpersonal perspective lead us to consider our evolving paradigms, paradigms that we have moved through during the 20th century, bringing us into the transpersonal phase of awareness for the 21st century. The clearer we can be about the paradigms which guide our practices, the clearer we can see that the issue is not primarily one of postmodern versus technical, but rather one of *different paradigms of thinking, worldviews and deep values and beliefs about our reality that impact on our life and work.*

When shifting into the postmodern transformative paradigm of transpersonal caring and healing, it seems that everything is being turned upside down. There is, however, an emerging order in the midst of the chaos, for all practitioners.

Kung (1982) observed that the paradigm shift does not necessarily include a destruction (or deconstruction) of all our values. What it does include is a fundamental ontological shift in values, from an ethic-free society to a society that is ethically responsible; from a technocracy which controls and dominates to technology which serves humanity. Such a shift is based upon a caring ethic and a spiritual vision for humankind and civilization. It is an evolution toward the quantum leap for humankind, a leap in which we are already caught, midair, trying to reach the other shore.

The Era III/Paradigm III postmodern 'leap' requires transformation within and without. As Lewis Mumford (1970) put it: all transformation begins and ends with self'. It is here, with self, that we are required to expand our reality and consciousness.

The transpersonal caring and healing model of Era III/Paradigm III is located more within a quantum framework than within conventional science. It posits transformative views and new premises of concepts such as consciousness, energy, intentionality, caring and reality itself.

9

Transpersonal caring–healing

We shall assume that, essentially, all energy is psychic in nature;
... this fundamental energy is divided into two distinct components:
a tangential energy which links the element with all others of the same
order (... the same complexity and the same centricity) as itself in
the universe; and a radial energy which draws it towards ever greater
complexity and centricity—in other words forward ... we are
paradoxically led to admit that cosmic energy is constantly increasing,
not only in its radial form, but ... in its tangential one.

(Teilhard de Chardin 1959, pp. 64–65)

Transpersonal caring–healing premises
Energy, consciousness and caring: considering the quantum

... the higher level simply transcends the lower level ... it's immensely greater and
has an entirely different set of relationships.

... the lower level will be the enfoldment of the higher level, in another sense the
higher one contains the whole and the lower one is more linear. ... What is going
on in the full depth of ... one moment of time contains information about all of it
... the moment is timeless; the moment is atemporal; the connection of moments is
not in time, but in the implicate order.' (Bohm, in: Weber 1986)

Quantum theory in physics is considered to represent a fundamental principle of importance in relation to consciousness, intentionality, energy and caring. Within quantum theory, there is a radical departure from Cartesian dualism; it postulates the unitive principle of complementarity as one that may govern the interplay of matter and energy (Pelletier 1985, p. 55)—as Pelletier puts it, 'the apparent dualism of mind and matter can be resolved by considering it to be a matter of emphasis rather than the reflection of an ontological duality'.

Within the quantum, a concept of consciousness and living systems evokes an invisible, unknowable, subatomic universe. Pelletier (1985, p. 66) cautions that 'this is an ontological problem that cannot be resolved by more sensitive instrumentation; it demands a quantum leap to another level of explanation and theory'.

There is a tendency in Western thinking to consider consciousness and energy in nothing more than metaphorical terms (see Watson 1988a and Plate 4). Pelletier (1985, p. 59) points out, however, that this viewpoint is in direct contrast with Eastern traditions. Tibetan Buddhists, for example, believe that thought is infinitely powerful and actually holds sway over matter. Quantum physics is increasingly lending credence to this notion, in that infinite energy can be an attribute of an infinitely short wave of vibration—that is, energy as ascribed to thought processes helps to make new understandings of mind–body interactions. For example, if, even metaphorically, consciousness carries energy, then new explanatory modes emerge for phenomena such as prayers, healing at a distance and one's caring consciousness in a given moment.

Within these emerging science views, our perspectives of appearance and reality are totally reordered. Quantum thinking per se deals with both the complementary and contradictory aspects of life; the paradox of the ordered and chaotic way in which the world works. The quantum perspective accommodates the rapid changes we are experiencing within the postmodern era, and these have little resemblance to what we have known before.

More specifically, quantum theory deals with *both particles and matter* that are *localized* in time and space, and also with *energy matter* that is *wave like*, spread out and *non-localized*. Particle and wave phenomena are two very different ways of looking at the world. However, the paradox is that they are simultaneously present, as contradictory yet complementary realities.

Quantum physics and quantum mechanics are concerned with what lies behind the appearances of matter, form and the particle-like material world. The notion of quantum introduces the concept of field as waves that are spread out. In principle, a field within this paradigm extends throughout the universe.

Newman (1994) uses aspects of the holographic model as part of her theory of health as expanding consciousness. She and others have used the 'two pebbles in the water' image to illustrate the quantum wave movement. As two pebbles are thrown into water, the waves radiate toward each other. They meet and interference patterns evolve, spreading throughout and becoming a part of the whole of each previous pattern.

Physicist Nick Herbert (1994) uses the metaphor of 'backstage/center stage' as a way to explain scientific reality based upon Heisenberg's 'uncertainty principle' (1927). In this framework of 'center stage' thinking, there is an 'actuality' and appearance that makes it appear that reality is localized; the appearance one sees is manifest as ordinary mass and particular matter. In the manifest world (*center stage* reality), we see the world as localized, separate and particle-like. *Backstage*, however, there is the 'possibility' waiting to be brought to actuality. It is here within the 'backstage'possibility that the quantum field is wave-like and everything is connected. At this 'backstage' level, the matter and energy of the universe are 'wave like' possibilities that depend upon observing, looking, participating and dialoguing with the universe. This process carries with it a degree of intentionality and freedom of choice.

At the 'backstage' level, we are co-creating reality within the quantum, complexity, chaos models of thinking (see p. 107). Other contrasts that can be made in addition to appearance and reality, center stage and backstage, are:

- direct/indirect
- explicit–actual/implicit–potential
- visible/invisible
- explicative/implicative order.

There is something 'infinitely beyond' that requires insight, apprehension beyond language, new images and pursuit. New models of science are making room for spirit. As philosopher Hans Kung (1982) put it: 'the standard answer to "Do you believe in spirit?" used to be, "Of course not, I'm a scientist". This is fast becoming "Of course I believe in spirit. I'm a scientist"' (in: Wilber 1982, p. 4).

Karl Pribram, who as a basic neuroscientist used the image of the brain as a hologram, predicted as far back as 1977 that the soft sciences of today would be the core of hard science in 10 to 15 years time. He predicted the emergence of a clear holism that would encompass all of science. Much of this is moving forward as he predicted.

Fundamental to all of these postmodern models is the quantum notion of connectedness. As Bohm (1988) puts it: 'we have overlooked the most fundamental question of reality and the universe ... the notion of *unbroken wholeness—the interconnectedness of all things.*' Bohm proposed consciousness as residing in the implicate order, whereby it eventually manifests in some explicate order— that is, consciousness is a more subtle form of matter and movement. He invoked a holographic notion to suggest that, in a holographic movement, there is no separation of space and time. If we seem separate, we are adhering to the manifest world as the basic reality. Within the non-manifest world of quantum physics, however, reality is all interpenetrating and interconnected as *one*: 'so we say, deep down, consciousness of (human) kind is *one* … If we don't see this, it is because we are blinding ourselves to it' (Bohm 1988).

Quantum caring field: holographic caring moment

This section relates the concepts of quantum and hologram to caring and healing, and draws heavily upon my earlier work (Watson 1987, 1988a, b). I have used the notion of a caring field to convey the quantum concept of waves radiating from each person and becoming part of a new field of possibility, all within a caring moment, affected by one's consciousness and intentionality (Watson 1988a, b)

The thinking from quantum physics and holographic models of science evokes new metaphors and a new aesthetic language to reflect some of the metaphysical and human dimensions of transpersonal caring, consciousness and energy. The holographic metaphorical model of science suggests a new wholeness in all the parts and a perspective wherein consciousness is more nearly cause than effect (Battista 1982, Bohm 1988, Harman 1982, 1987a, b, Pribram 1982, Wilber 1982). As Harman (1982, p. 139) explains, the 'old' science attempts to explain away consciousness, rather than understand it. The holographic theory suggests consciousness as a pulse of energy which in the physical domain seems to occur at a particular instant in time, while in the frequency domain it is 'timeless, eternal, and beyond time and space'.

Some of the recent work in physics and neuroscience speculates that the brain, and indeed the universe, may be like a hologram. A hologram (Plate 5) is described as having a realm of frequencies and a potential, underlying illusion of connections—e.g. the whole connection is in each part, although it can't be seen as such in illusionary worlds (Watson

1987). Pribram (1982) suggests that humans construct 'hard' reality by interpreting frequencies from a dimension transcending time and space. Contemporary nursing theoretical systems (Newman 1992, Parses 1981, Rogers 1970) accommodate holographic thinking by defining human beings as energy fields: open systems engaged in continual energy exchange with the environment, centers of energy, patterns of consciousness and so on. An energy field of consciousness is a non-physical phenomenon (Weber 1982).

A science of cells, at a less sophisticated stage of evolving science, considers physical causation to be somehow more 'real' than the more abstract levels of energy field or field-consciousness. Higher-order concepts, introduced in transpersonal caring–healing processes, invoke an expanded science model.

Fundamental issues related to ontologies, epistemologies, values, worldviews and intentions are now being questioned and clarified to address future directions for nursing science. Within the Era III/Paradigm III transpersonal caring–healing model proposed here, a hologram provides a new science language, as well as a new gestalt for viewing the transpersonal, caring–healing, human field-consciousness phenomena.

Some of the basic principles within holographic thinking include the following (Watson 1988a):

- The whole is in the part.
- There is an inseparable interconnectedness between humans and between humans and the universe.
- Mind/consciousness is joined; consciousness is communicated.
- Human consciousness is spatially extended; consciousness exists through space.
- Human consciousness is temporally extended; consciousness exists through time.
- Non-physical consciousness is dominant over physical matter.

In applying the hologram metaphor to the transpersonal, caring–healing paradigm, one can consider the following Era III/Paradigm III transpersonal caring–healing framework (after Watson 1987, 1988a):

- The whole caring–healing consciousness is contained within a single caring moment.
- The one-caring and the one-being-cared-for are interconnected; caring and healing are connected to other humans and to the higher/deeper energy of the universe.
- Human caring–healing processes (or the non-caring, non-healing consciousness of the nurse or other practitioner) are communicated to the one-being-cared-for.
- Caring–healing consciousness is spatially extended; such consciousness exists through space.
- Caring–healing consciousness is temporally extended; such consciousness exists through time.
- Caring–healing consciousness is dominant over physical illness and treatment.

Such thinking, related to caring consciousness and energy, is consistent with Dossey's notion of non-local consciousness. It allows us to go beyond the physical matter orientation of reality and healing.

Consider Zukav's (1990) views of the relationship between consciousness, energy and light. They allow us to reconsider the power of our caring–healing consciousness and its relationship to energy, transcendence and Era III/Paradigm III thinking:

- A thought is energy, or light, that has been shaped by consciousness. (p. 105)
- Emotions are currents of energy with different frequencies. Emotions we think of as negative, such as hatred, envy, disdain and fear, have a lower frequency and less energy than emotions that we think of as

positive, such as affection, joy, love, compassion (and caring). When you choose to replace a lower-frequency current, such as anger, with a higher-frequency current, such as forgiveness (caring, love), you raise the frequency of your light. (p. 94)

- Different thoughts create different emotions. Thoughts of vengeance, violence and greed, or thoughts of using others, for example, create emotions such as anger, hatred, jealousy and fear. These are low-frequency currents of energy, and therefore they lower the frequency of your light, or consciousness. (Creative or loving or caring thoughts invoke higher-frequency emotions and raise the frequency of your system.) (pp. 94–95)

- Lower-frequency systems pull energy from higher-frequency systems. If you are unaware of your emotions and thoughts, your frequency will be lowered by (you will lose energy to) a system of lower frequency than your own. (p. 95)

- If your thoughts are thoughts that draw low-frequency energy currents to you, your physical and emotional systems will deteriorate and emotional and physical disease can follow.

- Thoughts that draw higher-frequency energy currents (light and higher consciousness) will create physical and emotional health.

- A system of higher-frequency will soothe, calm and refresh you because of the effect of the quality of its light upon your system. Such a system is 'radiant'. (p. 95)

- When you choose to allow higher-frequency currents of energy to run through your system, you experience more energy. (p. 94)

- By choosing your thoughts, and by selecting which emotional currents you will release and which you will reinforce, you determine the quality of your light. You determine the effects that you will have upon others, and the nature of the experiences of your life. (p. 94)

- When you release a negative thought, or a negative feeling, you release lower-frequency currents of energy from your system and this, literally, allows an increase in the frequency of your consciousness. (p. 96)

- Light represents consciousness. By choosing our thoughts and awakening to our consciousness we reinforce and determine the quality of our light. You/we can determine the nature of the experiences of our life. (pp. 94–95)

- If we are aware of the light of our spirit (soul) consciousness, we are able to expand our awareness and reach to a higher level of existence. (p. 95)

(Reprinted with the permission of Simon & Schuster, Inc., from 'The Seat of the Soul' by Gary Zukav. Copyright © 1989 by Gary Zukav.)

These emerging ideas of hologram, quantum, consciousness and energy provide a new union between science and metaphysics (Harman 1991). They incorporate consciousness as evolving, and consciousness and energy as one; we can select our thoughts and consciousness by becoming more aware of this way of thinking.

The Era III/Paradigm III allows for both immanence and transcendence. With respect to caring, 'a single caring moment becomes a moment of possibility' (Watson 1989). When two people enter into a caring moment, a new field of consciousness, of possibilities, is created. Both can share consciousness or tap into another field, the universal energy field or universal spirit, which in turn has healing possibilities and recreates wholeness and 'being in the right relation' (Quinn 1996) at multiple levels.

The coming together within a transpersonal caring–healing context, viewed within the holographic framework, can provide an avenue for shared consciousness between the one-caring and the one-being-cared-for (Overman 1986). The caring–healing moment transforms from a two-field to a one-field consciousness. In the transpersonal caring framework proposed, both the one-caring and the one-being-cared-for are co-participants in the process that can potentiate self-healing, regardless of the medical condition. In such a transpersonal caring moment, both are capable of transcending time, self and space.

As Whitehead (1953) described it, this shared caring experience creates its own field (Fig. 9.1). His notion of concrescence indicates the coming together of many to form one. He explained that all past experiences are brought to bear on present occasions and merge to form the current experiences. Concrescence and the notion of transpersonal caring–healing imply a completion or a wholeness in the formation of the one-caring and imply the intersubjectivity and interconnectedness of persons and the universe.

While such holographic thinking associated with caring–healing consciousness does not dictate specific behaviors or actions; the caring–healing consciousness, held as an intentionality and moral ideal during a transpersonal caring moment, directs the nurse and other health practitioners toward new ontologies and epistemologies in developing postmodern theory and postmodern nursing science and beyond.

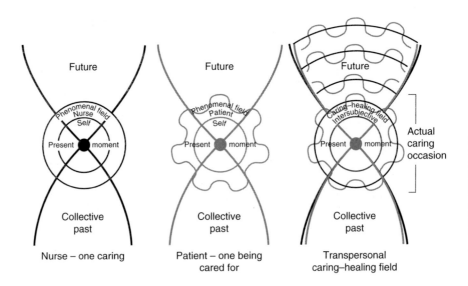

Figure 9.1 The caring field and caring moment. (From 'Nursing: Human Science and Human Care' by Jean Watson © 1988 Sudbury, MA: Jones and Bartlett Publishers, www.jbpub.com. Reprinted with permission.)

The transpersonal caring moment
(after Watson 1988a, pp. 58–59)

Transpersonal refers to an intersubjective, human-to-human relationship, which encompasses two individuals in a given moment, but simultaneously transcends the two, connecting to other dimensions of being and a deeper/higher consciousness that accesses the universal field and planes of inner wisdom: the human spirit realm.

At its core, transpersonal recognizes that the power of love, faith, compassion, caring, community and intention, consciousness and access to a deeper/higher energy source, i.e. one's God, is as important to healing as are our conventional treatment approaches, and is possibly even more powerful in the long run.

At its root, transpersonal caring honors the unity of being, shifting levels of consciousness. It seeks to harmonize *being* for self and other in relation to one's deeper/higher self in the world. In this model, then, a transpersonal caring moment may also become the field which manifests the space between us and the universe, the transpersonal space (Lawlis 1996).

In this way of thinking about a holographic model of caring, transpersonal caring and caring relations are those scientific, professional, ethical, yet aesthetic, creative and personalized giving/receiving moments between two people that allow for contact between the subjective world and consciousness of the two. Transpersonal occurs from person to person, but goes beyond either individual. This caring moment can release inner power and strength and help the person to gain a sense of inner harmony. A caring moment generates and potentiates the self-healing processes by facilitating access to one's own inner healer, while simultaneously going beyond self and opening up access to a wider universe (Dossey 1984).

In this framework, the two individuals who come together in a caring moment are both in a process of being and becoming. Both individuals bring with them to the relationship a unique life history and phenomenal field (i.e. a field that is uniquely experienced by/from the inner life world of each), and both are influenced by the nature of the moment, for better or for worse, depending upon the consciousness, intentionality and authentic being of the one-being-cared-for. As the two come together, the two separate individuals create a new field. Both are part of this new whole, in the moment, and this moment in turn becomes part of the life history of each person.

A caring occasion (after Watson 1988b, pp. 58–59)

Two persons coming together in a caring encounter within their unique life histories and phenomenal fields comprise an *event+*, or *actual caring occasion* ('event+' is based upon Whitehead's 1953 notion of event or actual occasion.) When two come together in a given moment, an opportunity, an actual occasion for human caring, is created. This moment is a focal point in space and time in which experience and perception take place, but the actual moment has a field of its own that is greater than the occasion and the moment itself. As such, the process can go beyond itself, yet arise from aspects of itself that become part of the life history of each person, as well as part of some larger, deeper, higher, complex pattern of life. This notion of the moment being present, in actuality, but also being transcendent and beyond the moment, is part of the understanding of the concept of transpersonal: beyond self and beyond the moment, yet containing both.

An *actual caring occasion* or *transpersonal caring moment* involves action and choice by both the one-caring and the one-being-cared-for. The moment of coming together in a caring moment, in a given occasion, presents the two with the opportunity to decide how to be in the relationship and what to do with the moment. Whatever is decided involves one manner and not another. If the caring moment is indeed transpersonal—it allows for the presence of the spirit of both—then the event of the moment expands the limits of openness and has the ability to expand human capabilities. It thereby increases the range of certain events that could occur in space and time at the moment, as well as in the future.

The transpersonal caring moment becomes part of the past life history of both persons and presents both with new opportunities. Such an understanding is based upon a belief that we learn from one another how to be human, by identifying ourselves with others or by finding their dilemma in ourselves, and by connecting with the universal human experience. What we all learn from this is self-knowledge and deep wisdom. The self we learn about or discover is every self; it is universal—the human self. We learn to recognize ourselves in others. This connectedness with other, and yet beyond self and other, keeps alive our common humanity. It helps us to stay connected with the human spirit, helping us to avoid reducing the human being to an object, separate from spirit of self and from the spirit of the wider universe.

In this kind of transpersonal caring moment or transpersonal caring relationship, the one-caring can enter into the experience of another, and the other can enter into the experience of the one-caring. This aspect of transpersonal incorporates a metaphysical, spiritual dimension, which transcends time, space and physicality.

Some of Whitehead's (1953) notions of concrescence (the coming together of many to make the one), in particular the notion that past, present and future are all contained in a given moment, are part of the explanation of a transpersonal caring moment. Bohm (1988, p. 207) also proposed that a moment of consciousness is a basic element which cannot be precisely related to measurements of space and time, but rather 'covers a somewhat vaguely defined region which is extended in space and has duration in time. The extent and duration of a moment may vary from something very small to something very large, according to the context (even a particular century may be a 'moment' in the history of humankind)'.

Figure 9.1 depicts the various components of transpersonal caring and a caring moment that transcends self, other, time and space, but holds past, present and future in the given moment in which they merge. In this framework, both the one-caring and the one-being-cared-for are co-participants in 'becoming' in the present and the future; both are part of some larger, deeper, complex pattern of life (Watson 1988b, p. 61).

The health practitioner engaging in this perspective holds a caring consciousness and intentionality towards wholeness as a moral ideal, not an interpersonal technique. In this model, one looks beyond the external disease per se, as presented by allopathic medicine. Transpersonal caring seeks deeper sources of inner healing, defined more in spiritual terms than disease elimination.

This transpersonal perspective entails a commitment to a particular end. The end is the protection, enhancement and preservation of dignity, humanity, wholeness and inner harmony. The transpersonal end also encompasses goals of self-knowledge, self-control, self-care and caring, and even the possibility of self-healing.

This notion of transpersonal is consistent with some of Newman's (1994) notions of consciousness. She writes about the nurse–client relationship in terms of forming shared consciousness: the interpenetration (or co-mingling) of the two fields. Within the postmodern caring–healing model proposed here, caring–healing consciousness becomes primary: a source and form of life energy, life spirit and vital energy which is connected to the energy of the universe, the universal energy field.

With consciousness posited as non-local (i.e. it is not localized in time or space or the body) it becomes what Dossey (1991) termed unbounded, unitary, one-with-all, infinite and omnipresent. A one-with-all, and all-in-one, consciousness allows us to reconsider transcendence as an expansion of self-boundaries, life perspectives, meaning, purpose, and non-physical phenomena, as well as of physical matter (Reed 1991, 1996).

Intentionality

It is helpful to give some consideration to the concept of *intentionality* and its relationship to the transpersonal dimension (Dossey 1996, McNeill 1987). Intentionality is not the same as the word 'intention', or as having 'good intentions'. The term *intentionality*, in the mind–body field, is a more technical, philosophical term meaning 'being directed toward a mental object' (Quinn 1996). Schlitz (1996a, b) defines intentionality broadly as 'the projection of awareness, with purpose and efficacy, toward some object or outcome. Philosophically, it is consciousness about something or some content of consciousness, such as belief, volition, expectation, attention, action, and even the unconscious' (Schlitz 1996b, p. 31).

As Rossman (1996) put it, when you declare your intention, it tends to mobilize whatever resistance is within you toward manifesting that intention. Schlitz (1996a, b) argues that intentionality sits at an interface between the subjective and objective points of view. From her perspective, a focus on intentionality allows one to chart the ways in which consciousness may directly and indirectly influence individual and collective well-being (Schlitz 1996, p. 31). Documented placebo effects could be considered evidence for conscious intentionality. For example, studies of the effect of hopefulness in cancer patient survival suggest intention at work (Olness & Mize 1996).

In this line of thinking, one also begins to appreciate the importance of belief systems and the spiritual perspective with respect to healing and consciousness. Levin (1993, pp. 54–56) put it this way:

> *Since the 19th century, over 250 published empirical studies have appeared in the epidemiological and medical literature in which one or more indicators of spirituality or religiousness, variously defined, have been statistically associated in some way with particular health outcomes. … This finding (i.e. religion is salutary for a wide range of acute and chronic conditions, morbidity and mortality) seems to hold regardless of how spirituality is defined and measured.*

Associated with this is the increasing attention to the role of prayer and healing. This has been popularized by Dr Larry Dossey through his well-known book, *Healing Words, the Power of Prayer and the Practice of Medicine* (1993). He surveys the field, emphasizing the possibility that prayer can influence health 'at a distance'. The study most often cited to support the role of prayer is the one by Byrd (1988) on coronary patients. A distantly located prayer group was randomly assigned to pray for some of the patients. These patients were matched against a control group of patients for whom there was no prayer. Byrd looked at objective indicators of well-being in the prayed-for group and the non-prayed-for group. He found that people who were prayed for by the distant prayer group, and who did not know that they were being prayed for, had fewer complications and left hospital more quickly. Other related studies are being replicated, while others have not been published in peer-reviewed journals. Nevertheless, Dossey, in particular, makes a strong case for healing words and non-local consciousness. In his view, prayer does not carry energy, nor is it sent via energy at a distance, but 'may simultaneously be present everywhere, enveloping sender, object, and the Almighty, all at once' (Dossey 1993, p. 84).

Clearly there are new and conflicting explanatory models emerging around these concepts and processes. The new relationship between caring consciousness, an intentionality of love and wholeness, for example, coupled with even the *idea* of thoughts holding different frequencies of energy (energy that thoughts both carry and communicate with others), helps to further envision a holographic model of caring consciousness, while also providing some new intellectual clearings for transpersonal dimensions of caring and healing.

Further, if consciousness contains energy, whether omnipresent and enveloping as Dossey suggests, or whether it is sent from a distance, in this model it becomes transcendent and 'non-local', rather than localized in the brain or body-physical. If this is the case, then Era III/Paradigm III thinking becomes all the more profound. New explanations of prayer, healing at a distance and other phenomena, previously unexplained by modern science but nevertheless occurring, now become more plausible.

This is truly postmodern thinking and beyond and takes us into the transformative cosmology proposed by Fox (1991) and Bohm (1988).

Considering consciousness and intentionality

Quantum theory suggests *true reality* is behind the *appearance* of separate, distinct entities, which are wave-like, oscillating possibilities, waiting to become actualities. The oscillating possibilities become actualities once we observe them, *look* at them, measure them and participate in seeing them with *intentionality*. In other words, at the appearance level, we see separate entities. However, those realities are only wave-like, oscillating possibilities until we intentionally look, to see. Then the possible reality becomes an actuality. We thus participate in creating reality, partially through our intentionality. Until we act on the possibility, it remains a possibility, not an actuality.

This line of thinking related to intentionality connects with the concepts of *consciousness, energy* and *light* discussed by Zukav (1990) and, described earlier in this chapter. For example, if our conscious intentionality is to hold thoughts that are caring, loving, open, kind and receptive, in contrast to an intentionality to control, manipulate and have power over, the consequences will be significant for our actions. The consequences can be seen to be based on the different levels of consciousness, the intentionality and the energy vibrations that are associated with the different thoughts.

Within this quantum paradigm of complexity, chaos and non-linearity, non-local consciousness and intentionality can be seen as wave like, with 'backstage' possibilities (Herbert 1994; see p. 107) awaiting to be brought into actuality by the co-participation of the consciousness and intentionality of the one looking. If consciousness is wave like with connections 'backstage', it also transcends time and space.

Another characteristic within the new quantum reality for caring is the notion of quantum ambiguity. Ambiguity and quantum ambiguity involve an entirely new way of thinking about reality. A quantum uncertainty exists; this ambiguity and uncertainty are affected by concepts of intentionality, which are affected by choice and options within the consciousness of the participant.

Herbert (1994) describes quantum ambiguity as a deep, almost inexpressible ambiguity in a world of possibilities and potentialities. One's consciousness, one's intention and one's participation in the so-called 'quantum magic soup' is what contributes to actual reality; when we look with intentionality, then we 'unambiguate the soup' and actualize the wave-like possibilities. Once one chooses and acts, the possibility becomes actualized.

The notion of ambiguity in human relations and human consciousness provides a richness of life and a new sense of freedom and choice. To see this moment as not moving, as if according to a law, predictably into the next moment is a sense of freedom in and of itself, but in quantum ambiguity this becomes true, a revolutionary sense of dynamic being, living and life itself.

This line of postmodern and beyond thinking holds powerful implications for a moment of caring and for considering a transpersonal caring moment. The radical quantum reality for caring suggests that this moment is not a moment of actuality but a moment of possibility.

Harman (1991) and others have proposed this 'backstage' order of moments of possibilities as a higher order that is full of wholeness with more energy, more insights and more potentialities, while containing the lower level within it. In his framework, Bohm (1988) refers to the super-implicate quantum theory order as an alternative to the current modern, narrow, Western epistemology.

The implicate order unfolds and is not determined by time and space as we know them. There is what Bohm (1988) refers to as the creative play of the universe. From its deep recesses (backstage), the universe evokes different combinations; it is unfolding, developing and flowering (Sperry 1987). The metaphor of the acorn and the oak tree captures some of the notions of the quantum: the implicate, explicate unfolding order. For example, the acorn contains all the oak tree within itself; it is 'backstage', so to speak, with potentialities and ambiguities awaiting to unfold and bring into material manifestation the actuality of the oak tree.

Consciousness is considered a more subtle form of energy, matter and movement; it is grounded in something infinite. Harman (1991) suggested that in higher states of consciousness (such as healing), there is an awareness of being with the universe and all its creatures, of a knowing beyond matter and actualized reality; a form of gnosis (intuitive/spiritual knowledge). This notion of consciousness and intentionality evokes a creative, intuitive, spiritual dimension which is not limited in the way we might expect the mind to be limited within the modern thinking of mind as localized and residing in the brain.

Considering transpersonal consciousness and intentionality in mind–body research

Consciousness is considered an epiphenomenon in medical and psychology literature. Recent developments in mind–body research have paid little attention to the possibility that people can consciously and deliberately (intentionally) use thought, images and feelings to influence their physiology and physical health. Nevertheless, this area is becoming more advanced as new explanatory models, such as quantum notions, emerge.

Other developments involve concepts such as *subtle biological energy*, even though it has not as yet been confirmed by conventional science (Benor 1996). Evidence for this kind of energy can be found in sensations of heat, tingling, cold and so on, as perceived by healers and those being healed during healing; changes in the energy fields can be felt by therapeutic touch practitioners in scanning the bodies of those being healed. Other evidence is related to sensations before and after healing sessions.

More specific to caring consciousness and intentionality are studies reported by Watkins (1996) showing how negative emotions, such as anger, were found to significantly impact left ventricular function (Ironson et al 1992) and 5-year mortality post-infarction (Denollet et al 1996). Watkins (1995, 1996) also pointed out that there has been a whole range of negative emotions that have been shown to modulate immunity. Even more interesting is his suggestion that, in order for a therapeutic touch practitioner to be effective and produce physiological change, *the practitioner must have the positive intention to heal and a sincere caring feeling* (1996, p. 35, author's accent). He draws upon research from the Institute of HeartMath to explain why this is so: 'the feelings of care generate coherence in the electromagnetic fields radiated by the heart'. He also reports that the institute has developed new techniques to assess how well the electromagnetic fields can be measured.

The purpose here is not to quote extensive studies, but to point out that there is increasing attention to undertaking research that ties these concepts of caring, intentionality and energy together. Watkins (1996, p. 35) tries to distinguish between mindful intentionality, such as visualization and positive affirmations, 'which produce only minor physiological effects. In contrast, intentionally shifting the emotions into a positive state by focusing on the heart and sincerely re-experiencing feelings of care and appreciation, can produce sustained physiological changes'.

In this paradigm, the postmodern body resides in consciousness, rather than consciousness residing in the body. The postmodern quantum body will be discussed further in the next chapter but, in this line of thinking, consciousness is non-localized and transcends time, space and physicality; there is a dimension of unbroken wholeness and connectedness within the field of universal consciousness, within which the body physical resides (see also Ch. 11).

The Era III/Paradigm III framework takes us beyond the modern masculine archetype, and beyond mechanical, sterile, strict rationalist, objectivist and body-physical practices which have become all too common. It is here that 'transpersonal caring–healing' becomes most actualized within a new model, or cosmology, although some aspects of transpersonal caring–healing obviously can and do occur within the other modern practices of Era I and II/Paradigm I and II.

Newman (1994) points out that the third paradigm of unitary consciousness (with its origin in Rogers,1970) incorporates the old paradigm, but transforms it. The new can retain the phenomena of the old, but explain and understand the phenomena from a different standpoint. The expanding Era III/Paradigm III presents a broader, more complex and more complete explanation of phenomena which, viewed from a new vantage point, will have entirely new meaning.

The postmodern and beyond paradigm embraces caring consciousness and unitary connectedness of all, actually helping to transform the modern medically dominated paradigm, whereby technology, science and practitioners are transformed within the new. It is here, in transpersonal caring–healing Era III/Paradigm III thinking, that holographic images and metaphors of quantum can be understood as one emerging models of science, of the brain, of consciousness and, indeed, of the universe.

For example, quantum theory and complexity science are now posited as the science and new cosmology that can help show the way to the 21st century, moving us past our staid and set mechanical universe. Whether considering quantum theory, or holograms or complexity theory, the fundamental idea is that all things in nature are interrelated and organize themselves into patterns.

In complexity theory, it appears that patterns are chaotic, with a complex non-linear order and unpredictable behaviour. In complexity and quantum science models, scientists are seeing the future as open; we are all called to participate in a new dialogue with nature and the higher order of the universe. Rather than sustaining a fixed view of the universe as controllable, objective, predictable and ordered, the latest views and emerging cosmology within the postmodern discourse involve a perspective that invites spontaneity, uncertainty and unpredictability.

This perspective is fundamental in bringing about a new order of the universe as complex, dynamic, interdependent, open and changing. The process is non-linear and appears chaotic or random but, in the margin, or on the edges of the evolving systems, there are forces of reciprocity between order and chaos, where new forms of order emerge. Within a new consciousness, creativity exists in the midst of a set order, if one examines the points of turbulence—what Briggs & Peat (1989) call the turbulent mirror.

Within Era III/Paradigm III thinking, already extant in nursing and medical science, the world of caring consciousness and the concept of the human mind/consciousness is more quantum than physical. Caring theory and the world of transpersonal caring–healing allow us to consider a caring consciousness with an intentionality to care (and heal) as another context for postmodern nursing and beyond.

This emerging cosmology also holds moral and ethical dimensions. A caring consciousness model gives rise to moral issues and the contexts of human to nature interconnections, and human to human connections. Maxine Greene (1991) challenges us to have 'wide awakeness', that is, to become in touch with our own human landscape (unlimited possibilities, residing in quantum ambiguity). As educators, scientists and practitioners, Greene believes we should seek to shatter the paradigm through emancipatory self-reflective processes. We should seek to be engaged in 'futuring'—a going beyond, to what is not yet, but might be. She says it is our 'wide awakeness' of the moral ontological foundations that informs our cosmology and frames the questions about our epistemology, about the very nature of reality, of science, of caring, of knowledge and of consciousness. It is 'non-awakeness' that leads to a restrictive *one* path to caring, healing and knowledge.

Within the modern set, there was fixed reality; within the quantum, there is openness. In contrast to the quantum postmodern context for caring and healing, the modern resulted in a formula approach to people. It objectified, codified, re-ified and diagnosed human experience with 'official', modern, scientific knowledge'. This knowledge took on a separate life of its own, one that was disconnected; it had only one manifest reality (particle matter) and was unambiguous, with no room for paradigm shattering, futuring, co-creating or going beyond, to participate in quantum reality. It is in quantum reality that caring and consciousness take on entirely new meanings as we engage in dialogue with the universe.

Within and beyond our postmodern models, which are so free floating as we dismantle reality, we need a cosmology that allows for ambiguity, paradox, connectedness and freedom. We need a cosmology that allows creative participation in our dialogue with the universe and in co-creating an art of science. We need a cosmology that is metaphysically grounded in a moral ontology of caring and that embraces an epistemology open to multiple ways of being, knowing and doing. We need to seek and participate in the whole, even within a part; we need to evoke new possibilities within the actualities we envision. With this postmodern quantum reality, the world is not solid, real or independent from us, but exists in limbo between the real and the possible.

As Ray (1994) points out, 'the rise of the caring movement in nursing parallels the complexity (chaos and quantum) movement in modern science' (p. 25). She highlights the fact that concepts of complexity science are well represented in nursing literature. They include the shared concepts of relationality, belongingness, holism, value, purpose, choice, love and qualitative measures for seeing the movement of order, chaos, and change in the non-linear world. Consistent with the postmodern theme in this book, Ray points out that these views ground nursing firmly within the new science of complexity (quantum) and the new philosophy (and science) of consciousness.

Movement in this direction is consistent with Teilhard de Chardin's midcentury notion of the evolving consciousness of humankind, toward the *omega point* (Teilhard de Chardin 1959). Fox (1991, p. 51) says that the ultimate principle of evolution is not adaptation, but transformation—indeed a new cosmology (Bohm 1988).

The transformative consciousness, intentionality and energy connection, as part of a broader ethic and choice among health professions, offers new considerations and new awakenings to the nature of our being in a relationship with one who is in need of caring or healing. This deeper dimension becomes part of the transpersonal caring–healing paradigm—going beyond postmodern nursing and going even beyond nursing.

By integrating the feminine sacred archetypal spirit of women and nursing as part of one's way of being in relation with self and other (as part of one's conscious intentionality, to hold caring, healing and loving thoughts that offer wholeness), something else begins to emerge. There is a spiritual, if not sacred, dimension to transpersonal caring–healing work. Once one is aware of the power and direction of this evolution for self, for one's profession and even for humankind, it becomes even more of a personal process and challenge, if not a professional quest, to enter into this new space.

Summary of the transpersonal caring–healing model

Within the postmodern, transpersonal, caring–healing Era III/Paradigm III framework, the following basic premises for a postmodern transpersonal caring–healing model are made explicit:

- There is an expanded view of the person and what it means to be human—fully embodied, but more than body physical; an embodied spirit; a transpersonal, transcendent, evolving consciousness; unity of mindbodyspirit; person–nature–universe as oneness, connected.
- Acknowledgment of the human–environment energy field—life energy field and universal field of consciousness; universal mind (in Teilhard de Chardin and Bohm's sense of *mind*).
- Positing of consciousness as energy; caring–healing consciousness becomes primary for the caring–healing practitioner.
- Caring potentiates healing, wholeness.
- Caring–healing modalities (sacred feminine archetype of nursing) have been excluded from nursing and health systems; their development and reintroduction are essential for postmodern, transpersonal, caring–healing models and transformation.
- Caring–healing processes and relationships are considered sacred.
- Unitary consciousness as the worldview and cosmology, i.e. viewing the connectedness of all.
- Caring as a moral imperative to human and planetary survival.
- Caring as a converging global agenda for nursing and society alike.

Subsumed under these premises, as well as other principles from quantum theory and holographic images, we can generate new explanatory models for practice and research which serve as a guide to the postmodern nursing qua nursing model, which builds upon aspects of energy, consciousness and the ethical, moral and spiritual aspects of the ontological shift required for the future.

The next chapter addresses issues related to the evolving human. The ideas open up new vistas on how to consider and reconsider the transpersonal body, being and becoming.

10

The postmodern/ transpersonal body

Do you not know that your body is a temple of the Holy Spirit within you, which you have from God? (New King James Bible, 1 Corinthians 6:19)

I realised that if I remained in the hands of mainstream medicine, I would soon be dead, rather than diseased, meat. For conventional ... treatment was reducing me quickly to a body that was only material, to a body without hope and so without will.

(Kathy Acker, January 18, 1997, The Guardian Weekend, London)

One of my English colleagues confided in me that one of the exciting features of postmodern nursing and health was the way in which it allows us to reclaim the body. Yes, but for very different reasons than the conventional, modern approach. For when we shift towards a transpersonal model for healing, the body is no longer body-physical material, as object, but becomes a living, breathing subject. It becomes an embodied subjective world, a vehicle for one's ground of being, a reservoir of consciousness and embodied spirit. As William Blake put it: 'Man has no body distinct from his soul; for that called body is a portion of soul discern'd by the five senses, the chief inlets of soul in this age' (in: Murphy 1992, p. 2).

To reown the body in this age means we have to reclaim the soul. To consider that we have to reown the body, as embodied spirit/soul, may sound strange. We are so accustomed to firm boundaries between the mind, the body and the spirit, between the ego and the flesh, that at first it perplexes us to comprehend the body in so foreign a way.

Within this change in thinking from the modern to postmodern and the transpersonal, the individual unit of evolution is the soul, fully embodied yet beyond body-physical. We have been so split in our perception of physical–material versus non-physical–spirit, that we have only just begun to turn our attention to the needs of the soul in the latter part of the 20th century.

During the 20th century, nursing and medicine (as Kathy Acker high-lights in the quote above) quickly reduced a person to a body that is only material. This mindset has confined us to the separate five-sensory, body-physical human, focusing only on the body as object and the ego personality. The medical cure models generated from the rise of medical science have, with the best of intentions, sought to cure dysfunctions of the body-physical by controlling the cellular molecular level. They have been based upon external forces and external interventions. This type of conventional treatment can, and does, help to eliminate or fix body-physical ailments, but it cannot heal at the deeper, inner-healing, transpersonal level intended here.

An example of the conventional mindset in medical science and medical studies is the way in which one treats the body and sets up conditions to study the body. I recall a survey, undertaken as part of a national project related to medical education reform in the USA (Pew-Fetzer Task Group of Psycho-social Education, 1991–1992). As part of that project, some major medical schools in the USA reported their different approaches to introducing medical students to the human autopsy experience.

In one very prominent East coast medical school, it was reported that the learning experience began with the professor walking into the classroom, going to the chalk board and writing the words 'dead mammal' on the board. That was the students' introduction to learning about the human body. They began to learn about human life through the study of dead matter: the study of carcasses and corpses. This dead matter, however, had no spirit to teach about life. As Zukav (1990) pointed out, we cannot breathe intelligence and spirit into learning about life by taking human and animal forms apart in our laboratories. Some day, this method will be understood as a very primitive, if not barbaric, form of learning; there is neither consciousness nor spirit there.

Even traditional approaches to teaching about the body offer better ways than the 'dead mammal' approach. That same survey about medical education in the 1990s revealed other more enlightened options on how to introduce students to the study of the human body, even within the conventional modern paradigm. For example, while one medical experience began with the dead mammal model, another equally rigorous but more informed medical school, still on the east coast, began the same experience by having a candlelight memorial service. This candlelight service included faculty staff, students, members of the family and other loved ones. The service publicly honored the loved one(s) who had donated their bodies. Gratitude and appreciation was offered for the gift of learning about the human body and the mysteries of the body-physical. In this second learning experience, while still conventional, the human body was honored as the instrument of the soul; the donated body was treated as a gift, a sacred trust bestowed upon medical science for learning.

These two images, dead mammal and candlelight memorial service, capture the difference between modern, material, medical thinking and a postmodern, transpersonal perspective of the body. The latter approach is emerging from the margins of conventional medicine, even in the midst of the status quo. This shift, however, is relative and is still evolving. For, as Ken Wilber (1981) pointed out, most of us long ago lost our bodies, disconnected them from our ego selves, and disconnected ourselves from our soul and the spirit within. He insisted that we take the concept literally; he indicated that:

> I am almost sitting on my body as if I were a horseman riding on a horse. I beat it or praise it, I feed and clean and nurse it when necessary. I urge it on without consulting it and I hold it back against its will. When my body-horse is well-behaved I generally ignore it, but when it gets unruly—which is all too often —I pull out the whip to beat it back into reasonable submission. ... I no longer approach the world with my body but on my body ... My consciousness is almost exclusively head consciousness—I am head, but I own my body. The body is reduced from self to property, something which is 'mine' but not 'me'.
>
> (Wilber 1981, p. 106)

'Body' in the modern sense has been characterized by a plethora of competing and co-existing terms: 'disobedient, obedient, mirroring, stigmatized, sinful, postmortem, sanitized, angelic, desexualized, dangerous, dominant, dominating, deceitful, submissive, disciplined ... communicative' (Hickson & Holmes 1994). Other analyses of body have included 'the medicalized body, the disciplined body, and the talking body' (Hickson & Holmes 1994, p. 3). These notions of 'body' have been culturally conditioned with respect to modes of consciousness as well as body use.

Jackson (1989) referred to the 1970s, when studies of body movement and body meaning appeared in increasing numbers but were either overly symbolic or somatic. Such limitations in thinking suggested that the body could be reduced to the somatic, when in actuality the concept of 'somatic mind' mediates understandings and changes in which verbal consciousness plays little part. New transpersonal dimensions of the body seek to eliminate the dialectic and dualism between the body-physical and the metaphysical–spiritual, the immanent and the transcendent.

When considering the transpersonal postmodern body, we are invited to consider some ineffable questions, such as, 'Can cells think?'. Suddenly, the words of my Russian guide, 'You have touched me to the cells of my soul', take on new meaning. Suddenly, the words of the American writer and journalist Kathy Acker quoted above become more revealing when considering healing, hope and what lies beyond the body as a material object in the conventional medical world of treatment and cure.

William James (In: Murphy 1992, p. 231) framed an enlightened point of view consistent with a postmodern transpersonal orientation toward the body:

> *I have no doubt whatever that most people live, whether physically, intellectually, or morally, in a very restricted circle of their potential being ... much like a man (sic) who, out of his whole bodily organism, should get into a habit of using and moving only his little finger. We all have reservoirs of life to draw upon, of which we do not dream.*

James had a transpersonal vision, although it was not labeled as such. Within such a perspective, we are motivated to consider ideas that are not allowed within the normative modern medical framework. Other philosophers and sages across time have reminded us that we are embodied spirits, but also transcendent, something more than a physical–material body.

As we reconsider the body, we begin to see a sharp reflection and stark relief in the limitations of the modern body as machine, the body as material object alone. Within transpersonal postmodern considerations, it is suggested that the body is the lived body, an experience that could as accurately be called the lived self, because it precedes a distinction between body and soul, and between body and self.

Within the modern normative medical approach, therefore, the body-physical became the 'body-as-it', disembodied and separated from thinking, feeling, consciousness and experiencing. Such an orientation allowed us to have body parts repaired and replaced, becoming interchangeable, all at the external level, without consideration of the inner world of the body-as-self, as experience.

The limited modern view of the body, with its five-sensory existence, placed us as separate bodies alone in a physical universe. We sought to control our physical self and the physical environment. The modern world was considered unaccountable and unmanageable unless it was dominated, manipulated and controlled.

As Zukav (1990) said, we strive to dominate so we can survive; intentions have no effect; the effects of actions are only physical; matter is the only real entity. However, the emerging, postmodern, transpersonal views of the body shift to the internalized body as lived, experienced, and indeed transcended.

In the transcendent transpersonal view of body, the body remains fully manifest as physical, and certainly present in the material, objective world. At the same time, it also manifests itself as fluid like, as elemental vibrations of light and energy, as electrical currents. The body communicates and is in communion, beyond the corporeal surface. Each individual's energy field of consciousness is in continuous interaction and exchange with the whole inner and external environment, one's non-physical energy field of existence (see Plates 5–8). The mind, self, soul, spiritual and material are one.

The postmodern body then becomes the 'quantum body', the 'body electric', the 'multisensory–extrasensory body', the 'body-as-subject' (e.g. Hickson & Holmes 1994, Jackson 1989, Merleau-Ponty 1962, Murphy 1992, Zukav 1990). Within the transpersonal framework, the body becomes a living spirit, manifesting one's being-in-the world, manifesting one's way of standing in the world, and reflecting how one holds oneself in the world with respect to one's relation to self and one's consciousness (unconsciousness).

As Jackson reminds us, we are all familiar with examples and expressions of feeling 'uprooted', of 'losing one's balance', of 'losing one's footing', and of being 'thrown off balance'. In this model these are not just figures of speech, nor mere metaphors. This thinking represents the ontological postmodern shift in the transpersonal paradigm that I am proposing. It is an uprooting, or being off balance, in one's life or one's situation that is actually manifest in one's entire being and the body as a lived subject.

Jackson (1989) goes so far as to say that all of this is occurring in the cellular structural musculature of the body. The metaphors, such as our 'bodily standing in the world', actually refer to a 'basic ontological structure of our being-in-the-world' (Jackson 1989, p. 123). In this sense: 'uprightness of posture may be said to define a ... relationship with the world, so that to lose this position, this 'standing', is simultaneously a bodily and intellectual loss of balance, a disturbance at the very center and ground of our being. Metaphors of falling and disequilibrium disclose this integral connection of the psychic and the physical' (Jackson 1989, p. 123).

Metaphors of human movement, in this realm, do not symbolize reality; they *are* reality. The body re-emerges as Merleau-Ponty's (1962) 'body-subject', whereby we 'think through the body'. The body is beyond the five-sensory, body-physical, and is a vehicle of consciousness, a radiant being of energy and light, a multisensory, extra-sensory, holographic, quantum body-subject.

There is a cacophony of postmodern dis-courses about the body and human life itself. There are now voices and data from many fields, such as anthropology, sports, the arts, psychical research, comparative religions,

I recall a personal experience I had several years ago related to this modern-body-as-object moving to a postmodern-body-as-subject. I was participating in a Vipassana meditation retreat which required mindful attending to the body physical as experience. In doing so, I was confronted with the stark reality of how out of touch I was with my body as experience.

I had indeed treated my body as the horse, suggested by Wilber. My head–ego consciousness was separate from my body as lived. I discovered, through mindful meditation on the body itself, that there was much to learn. The pain, my own and others, absorbed and stored in the muscles and the cells, all became part of an embodied experience. It was a most painful awakening, It was only by meditating through the pain, with mindfulness and equanimity, and only by going through the experience itself, feeling the body and letting it speak to me, that I had a rude awakening to my own being, my own learning and my own inner teacher. That teaching and learning, that practice of mindful equanimity with self and body, continues to this day. Such self-practice and self-growth are neverending. Once one is aware of another way in which to consider the body and self, one begins to honor and tend to self, to transpersonal self, and to honor and regard another's body as a sacred vessel.

medical science, physics, technologies, and neuroscience. We can now identify extraordinary visions of most, if not all, of our basic body experiences, among them sensory–motor, kinesthetic, aesthetic, communicative, cognitive, consciousness and sensations of self.

Murphy (1992) points out that by listening to this cacophony of the postmodern discourse about the body and human life, we can harbor a range of capacities that no single philosophy or psychology (or biology) has fully embraced. The next section will reflect some of the cacophony of perspectives on the lived body, within the transpersonal realm.

The future of the body-as-subject

Michael Murphy's remarkable book *The Future of the Body* (1992), claims that the professional specialization of scientists and academic philosophers has contributed to the fragmentation of knowledge about the body and the human being. In turn, this has left us depleted and bereft with respect to aspects of transformation and the extraordinary possibilities available to us as embodied spirits that are capable of transcending physical, material life.

Drawing upon literature as one source of transpersonal awareness, I consider *Jane Eyre*, by Charlotte Bronte. At about the time Nightingale was writing *Notes on Nursing* (from 1848 to 1849) Charlotte Bronte was writing *Jane Eyre* (from 1846 to 1847). While Nightingale communed with her God and proclaimed the spiritual, non-physical realm as part of her reality, the notion of extrasensory communication with a realm beyond the physical was not accepted, unless it was within the religious experience of the day. Nightingale's 'calling' was from God, which was accepted in the religious context of the day. Not so for Bronte.

In the 19th century, critics derided the telepathic 'calling' messages which Jane Eyre received from Rochester one midnight, when he was a very long coach ride away. Upon hearing the voice of her beloved Rochester, Jane hurried to him the next day, even though she did not know where to find him. Charlotte Bronte both defended and explained the extrasensory experience by confiding in her friend and biographer, when he took exception to this unbelievable incident in the book, 'But it is a true thing; it really happened' (Afterword to Jane Eyre, Zeiger A 1960).

By such accounts, Charlotte Bronte believed in the possibility of communication at a distance, or extrasensory perception, at least for some finely tuned individuals. In order to further consider the concept of non-local consciousness, communication at a distance, or the notion of human(s) as multisensory or

Jane's experience
(pp. 422–424)

All the house was still; for I believe all except St John and myself were now retired to rest. The one candle was dying out; the room was full of moonlight. My heart beat fast and thick; I heard its throb. Suddenly it stood still to an inexpressible feeling that thrilled it through, and passed at once to my head and extremities. The feeling was not like an electric shock; but was quite as sharp, as strange, as startling; it acted on my senses as if their utmost activity hitherto had been but torpor; from which they were now summoned, and forced to wake. They rose expectant: eye and ear waited, while the flesh quivered on my bones. 'What have you heard? What do you see?' Asked St John. I saw nothing: but I heard a voice from somewhere cry:

'Jane! Jane! Jane!'
Nothing more.

'Oh God! What is it?' I gasped.

I had heard it—where, or whence for ever impossible to know! And it was the voice of a human being—a known, loved, well-remembered voice—that of Edward Fairfax Rochester;

and it spoke in pain and woe wildly, eerily, urgently.

'I am coming!' I cried. 'Wait for me! Oh, I will come!' I flew to the door, and looked into the passage; it was dark. I ran out into the garden: it was void. 'Where are you?' I exclaimed ... 'Where are you?' I listened.

... I seemed to penetrate very near a Mighty Spirit; and my soul rushed out in gratitude at His feet. I rose from the Thanksgiving—took a resolve—and lay down, unscared, enlightened. ...

I recalled the voice I had heard; again I questioned whence it came, as vainly as before: it seemed in *me*—not in the external world. I asked, was it a mere nervous impression—a delusion? I could not conceive or believe: it was more like an inspiration ... it had opened the doors of the soul's cell, and loosed its bands—had wakened it out of its sleep, whence it sprang trembling, listening, aghast; then vibrated thrice a cry on my startled ear, and in my quaking heart, and through my spirit; which neither feared nor shook, but exulted as if in joy over the success of one effort it had been privileged to make, independent of the cumbrous body. '

extrasensory being(s), you are invited to engage in the actual accounts of Bronte's story. Even though it was written over 100 years ago, I offer it now for reconsideration, but with new insights of human possibility.

Even though Bronte was writing in the 19th century about communicating at a distance, the phenomenon she conveyed is congruent with the notion of non-local consciousness and holographic quantum concepts: concepts such as extrasensory experiences and consciousness transcending time, space and physicality. These are experiences and phenomena common to humans across time, but which have been shunned by modern science.

In Bronte's time, as well as in the modern era, in spite of Bronte's assurance that the event absolutely happened, it was not believed. With new thinking, however, we can acknowledge that we are perhaps evolving from the five-sensory human into the multisensory and/or extrasensory human. Such thinking extends beyond body and environment as physical reality alone, to a much larger, dynamic system of which our physical reality is only a part.

The extrasensory human

As Zukav (1990) put it, the extrasensory human is able to perceive and to appreciate the role our physical reality plays in a larger picture of evolution, the dynamics by which our physical reality is created and sustained. His realm, however, is invisible to the five-sensory, body-physical-oriented person. Within the transpersonal view the invisible, non-physical is contained within the five senses, yet goes beyond them. The body becomes our conscious matter.

Murphy's (1992) work lays out the idea of these extraordinary dimensions of the body and personhood by focusing upon such elements as the perception of external events, somatic awareness, communication abilities, vitality, volition, sense of self and love, among others. It is through these that Murphy suggests 'metanormal' capacities: extraordinary types of embodiment.

He posits that all or most aspects of significant human development and evolutionary transcendence are produced by a limited number of identifiable activities, such as:

Rochester's experience, conveyed to Jane, later (pp. 450–451)

'I was in my own room, and sitting by the window, which was open; it soothed me to feel the balmy night-air; though I could see no stars, and only by a vague, luminous haze, knew the presence of a moon. I longed for thee, Jane! Oh, I longed for thee both with soul and flesh! I asked of God, at once in anguish and humility, if I had not been long enough desolate, afflicted, tormented; and might not soon taste bliss and peace once more. That I merited all I endured, I acknowledged—that I could scarcely endure more, I pleaded; and the alpha and omega of my heart's wishes broke involuntarily from my lips in the word—"Jane! Jane! Jane!"'

'Did you speak these words aloud?'

'I did, Jane. If any listener had heard me, he would have thought me mad: I pronounced them with such frantic energy.'

'And it was last Monday night: somewhere near midnight?'

'Yes; but the time is of no consequence: what followed is the strange point. You will think me superstitious—some superstition I have in my blood, and always had: nevertheless, this is true—true at least it is that I heard what I now relate. As I exclaimed "Jane! Jane! Jane!" a voice—I cannot tell whence the voice came, but I know whose voice it was—replied, "I am coming: wait for me" and a moment after, went whispering on the wind, the words—"Where are you?"

"Where are you?" seemed spoken amongst mountains; for I heard a hill-sent echo repeat the words ... I could have deemed that in some wild, lone scene, I and Jane were meeting. In spirit, I believe we must have met. You no doubt were, at that hour, in unconscious sleep, Jane: perhaps your soul wandered from its cell to comfort mine; for those were your accents—and certain as I live they were yours!

'Reader, it was on Monday night —near midnight—that I too had received the mysterious summons: those were the very words by which I replied to it. I listened to Mr Rochester's narrative; but made no disclosure in return. The coincidence struck me as too awful and inexplicable to be communicated or discussed.

From *Jane Eyre* by Charlotte Bronte (1960 edition)

- disciplined self-observation (mindfulness meditation)
- visualization of desired capacities (conscious intentionality)
- caring for others.

He suggests that all matter is elevated to the status of consciousness in that there is a sense of the transcendent spirit, the reverential and the soul energy which is made explicit as part of an emerging cosmology of unitary consciousness. These dramatic steps in exploring the future and current evolution of human nature and the body are congruent with Dossey's (1996) non-local consciousness views, and nursing theorists Rogers (1970) and Newman's (1994) notions of energy and consciousness. They are congruent with principles from the science of consciousness, holography and quantum physics. These emerging trends are within the transpersonal realm of meaning.

Even within the electronic and informatics media, and within interactional systems, we see the emergence of a different kind of human subject, in a different kind of social, human and technical milieu (Lather 1991). We now have airwave space, cyberspace, 'soft communications' and subtle energy concepts through the internet and virtual realities, which are now becoming the 'hardware' within the postmodern conditions of this era.

The space–time limits of messages, and the despatialization of work and communication, create new relations between author and text, between communicator and communication, between subject and object. In this new realm of virtual space and cyberspace, 'reality' is being constituted in the 'unreal', non-local, non-physical dimensions (Lather 1991).

Notions of human experience as a particular frequency range in the continuum of non-physical light is a concept that Zukav (1990) employs. He suggests that just because we cannot see light frequencies this does not mean they do not exist. He points out that we are all evolving within this complex universe. Indeed, Zukav maintains that the latest technological and scientific developments might be manifestations of our evolving consciousness into the non-physical realm of matter and energy. He suggests that the 'scientific accomplishments of our species reflect our awareness as a species of non-physical dynamics as they unfold within the arena of matter and time, within the realm of the five-sensory personality' (Zukav 1990, p. 130).

This postmodern transpersonal condition takes us beyond what we have considered the norm. Another literary example of the possibilities can be found in Oliver Sacks' book, *An Anthropologist on Mars. Seven Paradoxical Tales* (1995). He writes:

> *I am sometimes moved to wonder whether it may not be necessary to redefine the very concepts of 'health' and 'disease', to see these in terms of the ability of the organism to create a new organization and order, one that fits its special, altered disposition and needs, rather than in the terms of the rigidly defined 'norm'. For the norm is traditionally against a backdrop of pathology'.* (Sacks 1995)

Sacks' view of the extraordinary within the ordinary, the extra-sensory human potential that emerges when we transcend concepts of 'the norm', is consistent with Murphy's (1992) compilation of the evidence for human transformative capacity. Sacks spoke of the sensory 'consensus' by which:

> *... objects are heard, seen, smelt, all at once, simultaneously; their sound, sight, smell, feel all go together. This correspondence is established by experience and association. This is not normally something we are conscious of ... But we may be made conscious, very suddenly deprived of a sense or having gained one.*

> (Sacks 1995)

As Sacks reported, David Wright, the South African poet and novelist who was deaf from the age of 7, 'heard voices' as he watched a speaker's face. Sacks discussed Wright's experience as a neurologist and reported how Wright '"heard" speech the moment he was deafened; an anosmic patient of mine 'smelt' flowers whenever he saw them ...' (Sacks 1990, p. 6f).

Helen Keller is a familiar example of the sensory capacities that allow the human to develop extraordinary perceptual abilities. Murphy (1992, pp. 285–286) describes how Keller derived pleasure from touching works of art. Her description of 'touch' is quite humbling and can inform nursing and other health professionals of the deeper experiences that touch can evoke:

> *As my fingertips trace line and curve, they discover the thought and emotion which the artist portrayed. I can feel hate, courage, and love, just as I can detect them in living faces. The hands of those I meet are dumbly eloquent. The touch of some hands is an impertinence. I have met people so empty of joy, that when I clasped their fingertips, it seemed as if I were shaking hands with a northeast storm. Others have sunbeams in them, so that their grasp warms my heart. It may be only the clinging touch of a child's hand; but there is as much potential sunshine in it for me as there is in a loving glance for others.*

> (Keller 1954, pp. 100–110, in: Murphy 1992, p. 286)

Keller's extraordinary experience is not unique. Murphy (1992) discusses how the evidence for remarkable human capacities extends across such categories as:

- psychosomatic changes in abnormal functioning
- the placebo effect
- spiritual healing
- extraordinary capacities in disabled people
- mesmerism and hypnosis
- biofeedback training
- psychotherapy and imagery practice
- somatic disciplines, including:
    —the Alexander technique
    —autogenic training
    —the Feldenkrais method
    —progressive relaxation
    —Rolfing
    —sensory awareness work
    —Reichian therapy
    —somatic disciplines and integral practices.

Comprehensive research evidence for the transformative capacity of the human has been presented by Murphy. Some of the evidence lies outside medical science. It has been gleaned from research into adventure, sports, the martial arts, religious practices and Catholic saints and mystics, and from scientific studies of contemplative experience. Others, such as Brendan O'Reagan (1987), have summarized the evidence on healing, remission and miracle cures, providing additional scientific evidence of the human potential. This evidence takes us well beyond the modern vision of 'the norms' of the body, the human and human potential and, indeed, human transformation.

The authors point out that these experiences are found not just among the mystics, saints or extrasensory people with special capabilities, but 'dramatic transformations of mind and flesh are evident, too, in ... healing produced by placebos and prayer, and in many incidents of everyday life, and during practices that make only a partial claim on their practitioner's commitment' (Murphy 1992, pp. 542–543).

An emerging explanatory view of the postmodern/transpersonal body—the emerging human

One explanatory model of the postmodern/transpersonal body and human transformation possibilities is arising from new images of the body, its substance and functions, in the field of physics. Zukav's view is that we have to reconsider matter itself. He suggests we are leaving behind our exploration of the physical world as our sole means of evolution. He proposes that it is in the invisible or non-physical realm that the origins of our deepest potentialities are found.

He suggests that as we evolve beyond the five-sensory human, we acquire expanded notions of being. The introduction of consciousness is elevated to the evolutionary ontological process, whereby one's intention and attention shape experiences. As Zukav phrased it: 'What you intend, through the density of matter, through the densest level of light, becomes your reality' (Zukav 1990, p. 127).

In this line of thinking, we are reminded that all great teachers and sages across time have been, or are, multisensory or extrasensory humans. They spoke, or speak, to us and act in accordance with perceptions and values (conscious intentionality) that reflect the larger perspective of the universe—a universe in which we are never alone, a universe which is alive, conscious, intelligent and compassionate.

Within the non-physical realm Zukav posits, the consciousness and intentionality of the multisensory/extrasensory being exist in this invisible world. According to his line of thinking, the intention behind an action determines its effects. Every intention affects us and others, and the effects of intentions extend far beyond the physical world.

According to Zukav's framework, described in Chapter 9, a thought is energy, or light, that has been shaped by one's consciousness. All beings are systems of light; the frequency of our light depends upon our consciousness. When one shifts one's level of consciousness, one shifts the frequency of the light (Zukav 1990, p. 94). Within this physics model of light, energy and consciousness, emotions are considered to be currents of energy with different frequencies. Emotions we think of as negative, such as hatred, envy, disdain and fear, have a lower frequency and less energy; they are more dense, more 'heavy'. Emotions we consider positive, such as affection, joy, love, caring and compassion, have a higher frequency of light (Zukav 1990, p. 94).

According to this new thinking, when one replaces (or consciously chooses to replace) a lower-frequency current of energy (such as anger) with a higher-frequency current (such as love, caring and forgiveness), one raises the frequency of one's light. The different thoughts we hold in our consciousness create different emotions and different currents of energy. Emotions such as anger, jealousy, fear and hatred are low-frequency currents of energy which lower one's level of consciousness and lower the frequency of one's light. Creative, loving, caring and forgiving thoughts invoke high-frequency emotions of compassion and joy, raising the frequency of one's being. When you have higher-frequency currents of energy moving through your body, there is more energy.

Reconsidering caring and healing consciousness

This line of thinking has profound implications for the choices we make about how we wish to be and how we wish to live. As health professionals working with different emotional systems, we must be aware that 'lower frequency systems pull energy from higher frequency systems'. If we are unaware of our emotions, thoughts and consciousness, our energy can be lowered by, and we will lose energy to, another who has a lower frequency than our own. Zukav (1990) cites a common example. We speak of a 'depressed patient' or 'angry person' who 'drains' or 'sucks up' our energy. We are also aware of persons who soothe, calm and refresh because they have a quality of consciousness and light that affects our system positively.

Zukav reminds us that by choosing our thoughts and selecting our intentions through our consciousness, we offer different energy currents to ourselves and others, and determine the quality of our light in the world. We determine the effects we have upon ourselves and upon others' experiences in our life (Zukav 1990, p. 95), for consciousness represents 'light', and vice versa.

We can change the way we shape the light flowing through us by changing our consciousness by, for example, replacing a negative thought pattern, such as anger, with compassion; by choosing to understand, rather than judge. When one's consciousness shifts, the experience shifts. According to Zukav, every experience and every change in experience reflects an intention, through an informed awareness of choice and will.

As we learn to shape our light through our consciousness and intentionalities, we also learn to handle our energy and its depletion and replenishment. We do this by learning to connect with the universal energy to which we all have access. We can do this by acquiring a daily contemplative practice, such as breathwork[1], meditation or Tai Chi. Cultivating our own spiritual practices is one way in which to keep the energy flowing smoothly though our bodies; it is one way to seek to sustain a caring–healing consciousness and intentionality in the midst of complex and complicated systems, both human and institutional.

In reconsidering the postmodern/transpersonal body, we are simultaneously reconsidering what it means to be human. As health professionals, we are invited to awaken to the fact that all aspects of our energy, intentionality and consciousness affect our caring–healing practices, as well as our life experiences. If we awaken to this line of thinking, then we have to awaken to the fact that our spiritual journey across time and space is now affected by the quality of our light.

Such an awakening to our way of being represents a fundamental ontological shift for health professionals, and gives entirely new meaning to the power and possibilities of 'a caring moment'. This transpersonal perspective, within the postmodern project of being human, offers what Margenau (1987, p. 134) calls a dominant theme of 'human as spirit', which draws upon Huxley, Margenau and Zukav's view that the 'human in the universe is essentially consciousness in manifest form' (Margenau 1987, p. 134).

While it is important to acknowledge that this postmodern/ transpersonal view of body and person is still evolving, the shift is nevertheless dramatic. In this emerging view, 'the body is the instrument of the soul', as Zukav put it (1990, p. 188). Behind every aspect of health or illness of the body is the 'energy of the soul' (p. 189). The soul is not physical, yet it is the forcefield of our being. The higher/deeper self is not physical, yet it is the living template of the evolved human, the more fully awakened personality or professional (p. 91). Zukav's treatise on soul

---

[1]Cultivated, practiced breathing—attending to inhalation–exhalation; expansion and contraction of life itself; everything arising and falling away with each breath.

goes so far as to assert that your energy and influence radiate outward, soul to soul, through which you can become an instrument of constructive change. If you choose to focus your consciousness and intentionality on the strengths of self and others—on the virtues and on the higher self— rather than on others' faults and flaws, then you have higher frequency energy. Compassion, equanimity, loving, caring and forgiveness flow through your body and system of light, and flow to others.

It may now be proposed that, as a health professional, it is not possible for you to engage in healing work without coming to terms with your soul, your higher/deeper self, or without coming to terms with the existence of non-physical reality, the non-physical aspects of the human body and one's being-in-the-world. It becomes critical to be aware of one's consciousness, one's intentionality and one's authentic presence of being in a caring moment.

It has already been noted that within the modern, body-physical, five-sensory view of person and body, one is not aware of soul, energy, consciousness and intentionality. These are not recognized as being important for learning or for professional comportment. But, as professional models increasingly shift toward the postmodern transpersonal view, professionals and the public begin to evolve more consciously on the spiritual journey, whether in sickness or in health. We are moving closer to the spiritual, non-physical, inner, extrasensory realm to learn of the dynamic and creative energy currents of the soul's existence; to learn of the inner healing journey toward wholeness.

Soul work

If you embark into this transpersonal realm of caring and healing, which embraces the soul, and if you desire to know your soul, 'the first step is to "recognize that you have a soul". The next step is to allow yourself to consider: "If I have a soul, what *is* my soul? What does it want? What is the relationship between my soul and me? How does my soul affect my life?"' (Zukav 1990, p. 31).

This is part of recognizing the energy of the soul, of recognizing one's consciousness toward honoring it, and allowing the soul to infuse one's life. Zukav notes that to serve the energy of your soul is authentic power; allowing one's soul to 'shine through' is to bring it into the physical world and to hold a reverence for and love of life and all its mysteries. The soul perspective returns us to the archetypal, the sacred energy, the light of our being, which contributes to personal and human evolution.

Within the caring-healing professions there is now a call toward a deeper, transpersonal level of practice that demands awareness of an attending of the soul: one's own, and others. This practice awareness seeks to align self with soul. As such, this evolving, transpersonal human consciously invokes and receives the loving, caring assistance of his or her own soul and of other souls that it assists or that can assist it (Zukav 1990, p. 90).

Universal consciousness and the sacred unconscious

The Era III/Paradigm III, postmodern/transpersonal model of caring and healing turns the body and human being somewhat upside down. There is both an embodied consciousness and spirit and also a non-local, transcendent consciousness, which is capable of being connected with the universal sea of consciousness, across time and space. When one enters into this frame of thinking, one taps into what Margenau calls the 'sacred unconsciousness' (Margenau 1987, p. 132).

As we enter into this space, we are reconnected with the concept of the sacred archetype. In Jung's theory, the unconsciousness of every individual and the 'collective unconscious', the universal mind, are linked to archetypes (see Glossary of definitions, p. 285)—those mysterious agents that appear in many human situations but have no temporal or spatial connection (Margenau 1987, p. 132). This raises the metaphysical implications of health and illness, and of living itself. Using this model, one might posit that, for every physical illness, there is a metaphysical, non-physical counterpart.

Such thinking requires that, as health professionals, we pay attention to symptom as symbol; it is the soul trying to express itself through the body as a lived subject. Such thinking requires that we attend to myth, metaphor, meaning and symbols to understand what the body is expressing as a manifestation of the soul, as a vehicle of consciousness of the sacred, non-local unconscious.

As Jung, Margenau and others acknowledge, much of this inner healing approach embracing the soul goes back to the archetypal, the sacred unconscious. To quote Jung:

> The effective (numinous) potencies in the unconscious are the archetypes. By far the greatest number of spontaneous, synchronistic phenomena that I have had occasion to observe and analyze can easily be shown to have a direct connection with an archetype. This, in itself, is an irrepresentable, psychoid factor of the collective unconscious. This latter cannot be localized, since it is either complete in principle in every individual or is found to be the same everywhere. You can never say with certainty whether what appears to be going on in the collective unconscious of a single individual is not also happening in other individuals or organisms or things or situations.

(Jung, in: Margenau 1987, p. 132)

All of this points us toward Margeneau's (1987) and Houston Smith's (1982) notion of the sacred unconscious, which is that aspect which unites and connects us, soul to soul, with the archetypal, collective oneness. It is the non-physical ground of our being.

As Smith put it, to access true causes and motives, and supreme human opportunity and spiritual growth, one has to strike deeper still and become aware of the 'sacred unconscious that forms the bottom line of our selfhood' (Smith 1982, p. 178). The sacred unconscious in this instance is consistent with Zukav's (1990) notion of the soul. Within Smith's framework, sacred means to grasp life as if 'all things were one big miracle'. In this sense, he points out that the opposite of a sense of sacredness is not serenity or sobriety, but drabness, taken-for-grantedness and a lack of interest. It is the humdrum and prosaic (Smith 1982, p. 182). He called upon the belief that, as well as being a gift to be cherished, received and honored, life is also a task to be performed. The journey is towards the sacred unconscious, to touch that 'luminous mystery in which all things are bathed' (p. 184).

The paradox is that, on the one hand, we see how far we all are from the goal that beckons; on the other hand, in the Buddhist sense, there is no separation between *this* and *that*. We are already there. The Buddhist analogy of Indra's net of gems is already laid out before us: the universe is one great net, spread out, with at every joint a gem, and each gem is not only reflecting all the others, but is reflected itself in all. Campbell (1972, pp. 147–148) explained that we are all *one*: 'this is the *one*. We are experiencing it as an actuality, the unity of all … we include equally the past—our numerous, disparate, pasts—the present and the future, which is already here', like an oak tree already embodied in the acorn. Within this line of thinking, we are all bathed in the universal mind, the sacred unconscious, the oneness of all. Within this awakening, 'as human beings we are made to surpass ourselves and are truly ourselves only when transcending ourselves. Only the slightest of barriers separates us from our sacred unconscious; it is infinitely close to us' (Smith 1982, pp. 184–185).

The transpersonal caring model

In this transpersonal model, we have spread out before us a global image of an evolving humanity. To quote Margenau (1987, p. 135):

> *Human potentiality is limitless. All knowledge, power and awareness are ultimately accessible to one's consciousness. As a person becomes aware of the basic nature of reality (existence), he or she is motivated toward development, creativity, and movement toward the 'higher (deeper) self', and becomes increasingly directed by this higher consciousness. What is called 'inspiration' or 'creativity' is essentially a breaking through in ordinary awareness of these higher processes.*

> *Evolution occurs, physical and mental, and is directed by higher consciousness and is characterized by purpose. As humankind increases its level of consciousness, it participates more fully in this evolutionary purpose ... This view of man (sic), if it can be experienced by more than the small minority of persons who have apparently realized it through the centuries, would seem to provide the needed sense of direction and holistic perception and understanding which is needed.*

To engage in a transpersonal, caring–healing model involves transformation. A transpersonal self is a transformed self, beyond the ego self. Transpersonal, however, is different from transcendent, in that it is manifest in and through the person. While transpersonal means beyond the ego self and the personal, it does not deny the individual, and does not lead to a dissolution of a separate self.

In transpersonal caring, caring becomes both a moral ideal (Gadow 1988, Watson 1995) and an ontology. Transpersonal and consciousness also become primary in the process. A transpersonal caring relationship depends upon (Watson 1988a):

1. A moral commitment to protect and enhance human dignity and the deeper/higher self; the soul of the person is honored.

2. The caring consciousness of the nurse is communicated with the other on a level that both embodies and honors the other's physicality, but transcends the physical by preserving and honoring the embodied spirit; the person is not therefore reduced to the moral status of 'object'. There is then a connection between the persons, but also a new energy field is created by the consciousness and intentionality held in the moment.

3. A transpersonal caring connection is a focal point in time and space from which experience, perception and intentional connection are taking place. Such a caring consciousness and connection, one to another, has a healing potential. It is grounded in the individual experiences of the two separate persons, but goes beyond the two; the self connection is every self—the universal self. We learn to recognize ourselves in others by engaging in a transpersonal caring moment.

> Love alone is capable of uniting living beings in such a way as to complete and fulfill them, for it alone takes them and joins them by what is deepest in themselves. This is a fact of daily experience.   *(Teilhard de Chardin 1964)*

From ego self to transpersonal self

Since so much of the transpersonal/postmodern paradigm involves an ontological shift at the personal level, it is important to emphasize some of the characteristics that differentiate between the modern ego–body focus, to which we are so accustomed, and the transformative, transpersonal focus we seek for a caring–healing practice. The contrast between the two modes of being represents an ontological evolution through focused practice and one's self-development and spiritual journey. Through an on-going, contemplative practice and cultivation of 'mindfulness and equanimity with self and other', the characteristics of the transpersonal self become more manifest in our life and work. Table 10.1 presents the contrast between the different ways of being.

Table 10.1 Body–ego self and transpersonal self. (From 'The Inward Arc' by Frances Vaughn © 1986, 1995 2nd edn. Reprinted with permission of Blue Dolphin Publications, Inc., Grass Valley.)

Body–ego self	Transpersonal self
Ego centered	Ego transcendent
Judgmental/critical	Compassionate
Fearful	Loving
Opinionated	Wise
Intrusive	Receptive
Dominating	Allowing
Limited dimension of reality	Unlimited reality dimensions
Rationalizing	Intuitive
Controlled	Spontaneous
Restrictive	Creative
Closed	Responsive
Distant	Authentically present
Mindless/unaware	Mindfulness
Conventional	Inspired
Anxious	Peaceful
Defensive	Open
Separated	Connected-in-relation
Material world	Open to transcendent; spiritual
Self-closed	Self-disclosure
Unawakened consciousness	Awake
Worldview fixed, static	Worldview dynamic, evolving
Secular	Sacred

Notions related to the postmodern body and transpersonal human require an ontological shift in thinking about the body and the human being. These concepts, whether considered philosophically, metaphorically or scientifically, offer new understandings of personhood and of humanity itself, within the evolutionary scheme of the universe. These ideas are helpful in expanding our possibilities and our transpersonal consciousness, and for ushering in an emancipatory worldview for caring and healing practices and practitioners. The next chapter provides still another perspective of the body—from the world of metaphysical art, which considers the body artistically, as a sacred mirror.

11

The body as a sacred mirror

This chapter anchors some of the universal dimensions of the human as embodied spirit, in considering what it means to be human. It invites us to consider and reconsider the body from both a physical and metaphysical, artistic standpoint and, in particular, explores a series of paintings called *Sacred Mirrors* by Alex Grey (1990) (Plates 5–8).

'Sacred Mirrors' by Alex Grey

I first encountered this work in 1986 after hearing it reviewed on public radio. It was described as 'art for the 21st century'. The work and its description called out to me so much that I rearranged a forthcoming trip to the East coast to see the exhibit at the New Museum in Soho, New York. It was an experience to remember, and one that led me to contact Alex and engage him in my interest in his work.

Since 1987, I have used selected works from the *Sacred Mirrors* in numerous talks presented in the USA and around the world. Alex has also participated in a Summer Institute at the University of Colorado Center for Human Caring. The Summer Institute, entitled 'Caring and Art', was jointly sponsored by the Center and the Fine Arts Museum on the Boulder Campus of the University.

I have also had the honor to co-present my work on caring, with Alex, to a national nursing audience. It is a special pleasure to share Alex's work, through this book, with the broader nursing and health science community, even though many will have since become familiar with his published book (Grey 1990).

What is also unique about this work is that Alex Grey spent several years in medical school, studying human anatomy to enhance his keen interest in portraying the interconnectedness of body, mind and spirit. In addition to his work being exhibited in New York and in the University of Colorado Museum, it has also appeared in Boston; the University of California Museum of Art, Santa Barbara; the Chicago International Art Exposition; the London Regional Art Gallery; Canada; the Grand Palais, Paris; and the Sao Paulo Biennial, Brazil, as well as in numerous other exhibitions.

In this very special creative work of art, many physical and non-physical levels of the body are portrayed. The work is depicted as a 'graphic, visionary journey through the physical, metaphysical and spiritual anatomy of the self' (Grey 1990, Plate 5). The different images move from the detailed renderings of the body systems, each bodily system serving as a system of knowledge of its own (e.g. Plate 6). The series then progresses to images of the full-body-physical, capturing the three great races of the world, and the magnificence of all aspects of physical being.

From the body-physical onward, the series moves to the spiritual/ energetic level, envisioning the same law-like regularity of the metaphysical to mirror the anatomically correct details and regularity of the body-physical. At this metaphysical level, the art captures the sacred dimensions of being and the oneness of all. One can visually, artistically, metaphorically and even scientifically see the body as 'a living field of energy'.

If ever there was a vivid description of the body as being more than physical matter, Alex Grey's *Sacred Mirrors* is it. The work is considered so powerful by those who view it that it has been used, and most likely will increasingly be used, as an artistic, mental image to visualize and focus healing energy to various aspects of the body.

Consider the personal narrative that accompanies the art:

> The Sacred Mirrors *are a series of 21 images ... Each image is 46 by 84 inches and* *presents a life-sized figure directly facing the viewer, arms to the side and palms* *forward. This format allows the viewer to stand before the painted figure and* *'mirror' the image. A resonance takes place between one's own body and the* *painted image, creating a sense of 'seeing into' oneself. The* Sacred Mirrors *may* *be used as a tool to visualize and focus healing energy to particular parts of the* *physical and metaphysical bodies.* (Grey 1990, pp. 16–19)

As one views the many layers of the body artistically, one also sees how alike one is with others before and after the 'skin', and also how the skin separates one from another. We also see how the physical and metaphysical merge. This work cannot be depicted literally; it has to be experienced and realized as part of an awakening consciousness within the transpersonal realm.

As one can see from the metaphysical views, the art captures the yogic chakras labeled 'Psychic energy system' (Plate 7A) and the 'Spiritual energy system' (Plate 7B). The progression moves from the material world to the spiritual world. This movement conveys a process of transformation, from body-ego consciousness to spiritual consciousness. The psychic energy system offers an X-ray view of the body-physical and weaves together the non-physical and psychospiritual energy systems. Alex introduces what he considers to be a complex variety of energy systems and spiritual archetypes, which could be called the metaphysical aspect of the human being.

One of the strong universal dimensions of the art is the portrayal of the ancient Hindu chakra ('wheel') system of energy. The seven centers of energy are distributed through the body, from the base to the crown of the head (Plate 7A, B). Each center represents a different color and vibratory frequency. Beginning with the bottom, the base chakra is red (grounding).

Moving upward through the centers, the corresponding colors are: orange (sexual–creative); yellow (solar plexus–emotional); green (heart–love); blue (throat–voice); amethyst (third eye–transcendent); and white (crown–spiritual). As one progresses from the lower to the higher chakras, the energy vibratory frequency becomes higher and lighter. The colors blue, lavender and white are considered to be more spiritual colors, which means they have higher vibratory frequencies and are therefore lighter. The lower chakras carry denser energy and help to ground and center.

The idea is to have access to all the energy frequencies in order to keep oneself more balanced, whole and open. Through yoga and meditation, these energy points can be successively activated and release an ever higher/deeper realization of spiritual consciousness and bliss. Such experiences take us beyond the animal, instinctual level of existence, towards loving kindness, compassion and oneness with all.

Campbell (1972) noted that these centers are also known as lotuses; they are dormant until touched and activated by a rising spiritual power, known as kundalini. This power, kundalini, is a feminine Sanskrit noun, meaning 'the coiled one'. It refers to the idea of a coiled serpent, thought to be sleeping in the lowest of the seven body centers. In India, this power is considered to be a feminine, form-building, life-giving and supporting force by which the universe and all things are rendered animate (Campbell, p. 110). For a more complete description of the chakra system, Campbell recommends the textbook *A Description of the Six Bodily Centers of the Unfolding Serpent Power* (Shatchakra-Nirupanam 1931).

The aim in recognizing the chakra system is to 'awaken spiritually' by breathing energy and the breath of life into each of the seven centers in order to reach a deeper, higher level of consciousness, and a more inspired, alive and sacred existence. These ancient energy wheels or systems of energy are now commonly referred to in meditation and contemplative practices, and are acknowledged in healing work. In healing work, the centers are noted as needing to be 'cleansed', 'activated' and 'cleared'.

Carolyn Myss' work (1996) discusses the chakras as energy centers which depict sacred, ancient imagery related to the human. According to her research, the chakra system is an archetypal depiction of individual maturation through seven distinct stages, vertically aligned from the base of the spine to the crown of the head, suggesting an evolution toward the divine. Each stage offers a further refined understanding of personal and spiritual power.

Myss (1996, pp. 68–69) summarizes the spiritual life-lessons within the seven chakras as follows :

1. First chakra: lessons related to the material world
2. Second chakra: lessons related to sexuality, work and physical desire (and I might add creativity, and the birthing of something new)
3. Third chakra: lessons related to ego, personality and self-esteem
4. Fourth chakra: lessons related to love, forgiveness and compassion
5. Fifth chakra: lessons related to will and self-expression
6. Sixth chakra: lessons related to mind, intuition, insight and wisdom
7. Seventh chakra: lessons related to spirituality.

Within Myss' framework related to the chakra system, each of the seven centers directs us toward greater consciousness and spiritual evolution; indeed, she referred to these centers as the 'seven sacred truths'. The sacred truth, according to Myss, is that the power created by these archetypal forces transmits into our energy and biological system our interconnectedness with all of life and each other. 'All is One', is one way of honoring the fact that we are all part of the divine family. If we consider those who are different from us to be less than us, then we create conflict within our spirit and within our physical body. To work on the sacred truth that 'All is One' is a universal spiritual challenge.

While it is not the focus of this text, Myss goes on to present a model of the seven centers of the chakra system in which she synthesizes the ancient wisdom of three spiritual traditions: the Hindu chakras, the

Christian sacraments, and the Kabbalah's 'Tree of Life'. All of this system is referred to as the 'anatomy of the spirit,' which is also the title of her important work.

Table 11.1 depicts Myss' anatomy of the spirit tables for her notions of 'energy anatomy' which correspond with each chakra center.

The work of Myss takes the chakra notions to a deeper level of integration, while remaining consistent with Campbell (1972) and Grey (1990). Within this way of understanding the body and spiritual anatomy, posited to parallel the physical anatomy, understanding of the spiritual connections with illness grows, and we begin to know better how to be aware of and correct an energy imbalance in the seven sacred energy centers. This new/old understanding of the body helps us to see our embodied spirit and transpersonal/postmodern body in an entirely new light.

Another feature of Grey's art and narrative is its relation to the transpersonal, sacred feminine dimensions of existence developed throughout this book. The art of the sacred mirrors captures the concept of the unitary person, developed by Martha Rogers (1970), and now part of contemporary nursing philosophy and theory. This concept develops the interconnectedness between the human and the environment, and conveys a view of evolving consciousness. Grey's work artistically captures these contemporary nursing theoretical concepts, and offers a new clearing for considering theory and worldview shifts at the basic ontological level of being.

As he describes it, the *Sacred Mirrors* open us to the opportunity to see oneself in the fractured mirror of the material world. It is essentially the same world, but transformed—a world of unity and interrelatedness (Grey 1990, pp. 16–19). Referring to the narrative of *Sacred Mirrors*, Grey confides that the final mirror is an invitation to reflect on oneself and others as well as on one's entire surroundings as an aspect of God. Hence, sacredness of being, and the sacredness of all.

Table 11.1 Energy anatomy. (From 'Anatomy of the Spirit' by Caroline Myss © 1996. Reprinted by permission of Harmony Books, a division of Crown Publishers, Inc., New York.)

Chakra	Organs	Mental, emotional issues	Physical dysfunctions
1	Physical body support Base of spine Legs, bones Feet Rectum Immune system	Physical family and group safety and security Ability to provide for life's necessities Ability to stand up for self Feeling at home Social and familial law and order	Chronic lower back pain Sciatica Varicose veins Rectal tumors/cancer Depression Immune-related disorders
2	Sexual organs Large intestine Lower vertebrae Pelvis Appendix Bladder Hip area	Blame and guilt Money and sex Power and control Creativity Ethics and honor in relationships	Chronic lower back pain Sciatica Obstetric/gynecological problems Pelvic/lower back pain Sexual potency Urinary problems
3	Abdomen Stomach Upper intestines Liver, gall bladder Kidney, pancreas Adrenal glands Spleen Middle spine	Trust Fear and intimidation Self-esteem, self-confidence and self-respect Care of oneself and others Responsibility for making decisions Sensitivity to criticism Personal honor	Arthritis Gastric or duodenal ulcers Colon/intestinal problems Pancreatitis/diabetes Indigestion, chronic or acute Anorexia or bulimia Liver dysfunction Hepatitis Adrenal dysfunction
4	Heart and circulatory system Lungs Shoulders and arms Ribs/breasts Diaphragm Thymus gland	Love and hatred Resentment and bitterness Grief and anger Self-centeredness Loneliness and commitment Forgiveness and compassion Hope and trust	Congestive heart failure Myocardial infarction (heart attack) Mitral valve prolapse Cardiomegaly Asthma/allergy Lung cancer Bronchial pneumonia Upper back, shoulder Breast cancer

Table 11.1 (cont'd)

Chakra	Organs	Mental, emotional issues	Physical dysfunctions
5	Throat Thyroid Trachea Neck vertebrae Mouth Teeth and gums Esophagus Parathyroid Hypothalamus	Choice and strength of will Personal expression Following one's dream Using personal power to create Addiction Judgment and criticism Faith and knowledge Capacity to make decisions	Raspy throat Chronic sore throat Mouth ulcers Gum difficulties Temporomandibular joint problems Scoliosis Laryngitis Swollen glands Thyroid problems
6	Brain Nervous system Eyes, ears Nose Pineal gland Pituitary gland	Self-evaluation Truth Intellectual abilities Feelings of adequacy Openness to the ideas of others Ability to learn from experience Emotional intelligence	Brain tumor/hemorrhage Stroke Neurological disturbances Blindness/deafness Full spinal difficulties Learning disabilities Seizures
7	Muscular system Skeletal system Skin	Ability to trust life Values, ethics and courage Humanitarianism, selflessness Ability to see the larger pattern Faith and inspiration Spirituality and devotion	Energetic disorders Mystical depression Chronic exhaustion that is not linked to a physical disorder Extreme sensitivities to light, sound and other environmental factors

This view then raises new and ancient questions: 'If we are spiritual beings created out of divine substance, how does this suggest that we live? How does this suggest that we treat our bodies?'

Meditation for the transpersonal/postmodern body and self

Ken Wilber offers a meditation for the transpersonal self which is one suggestion as to how we might reconsider our bodies within the transpersonal sense. I offer it here for meditative considerations:

> I have *a body, but I am* not *my body. I can see and feel my body, and what can be seen and felt is not the true seer. My body may be tired or excited, sick or healthy, heavy or light, but that has nothing to do with my inward I. I have a body, but I am* not *my body.*
>
> I have *desires, but I am* not *my desires. I can know my desires, and what can be known is not the true knower. Desires come and go, floating through my awareness, but they do not affect my inward I. I have desires, but I am* not *my desires.*
>
> I have *emotions, but I am* not *my emotions. I can feel and sense my emotions, and what can be felt and sensed is not the true feeler. Emotions pass through me, but they do not affect my inward I. I have emotions, but I am* not *emotions.*
>
> I have *thoughts, but I am* not *my thoughts. I can know and intuit my thoughts, and what can be known is not the true knower. Thoughts come to me and leave me, but they do not affect my inward I. I have thoughts, but I am* not *my thoughts*

(Wilber 1981, pp. 128–129)

This meditation affirms that we are, or can be, a witness to our thoughts, desires and emotions, but our true self is beyond them. The transpersonal self allows you to go to the quiet depths of the soul, beneath the surface of the turbulent waves of the passing experiences, and connect with that which is timeless and eternal—the 'eternal moment' that Whitehead (1953) described.

In the narrative of *Sacred Mirrors*, the self is recognized as 'that which underlies, unites and directs the many physical and metaphysical systems. The *Sacred Mirrors* reflect the sacredness of the individual self, but also the unity with other people and cultures, and one's connectedness with the earth and the universe' (Grey 1990).

The *Sacred Mirrors* offers an artistic, metaphorical and metaphysical image for the postmodern/transpersonal caring–healing model. It conveys a sense of the sacred, the unity of all and the notion of evolving consciousness, an 'awakening from the body physical to an embodied spiritual existence'. Is such an awakening an expanded ontological awareness about what it means to be human, and what it means to *be*?

The following closing excerpt from Grey's work captures his own awakening and realization of his own truth of his body as energy and light (Plate 10):

I felt that my body was no longer just a solid, isolated object in a world of separate forms and existential anxiety, but more like a manifestation of the primordial energy of awareness that was everywhere present. The mystical experience is not some dreamy fantasy, as anyone who has had one can agree. Psychological research into the mystical experience has yielded the following definition: a sense of profound unity within oneself and with the outside world; a transcendence of space and time or a feeling of being in touch with infinity and eternity; a sense of sacredness, awe or numinosity; a sense of the supreme reality and truth of the insight; the embracing of paradoxes or transcendence of duality; ineffability; and overall positive affect.

The mystical experience is a transformative contact with the ground of being and, although it is beyond description, it gives people an expanded appreciation of life. During times of cynicism and despair, experiences that empower people to heal conflicts and choose life are especially valuable. I wanted my paintings to visually chart the spectrum of consciousness from material perception to spiritual insight ...

(Grey 1990, p. 31, with permission)

One last work of ancient art is included, to provide a visual representation of the transpersonal body and consciousness. This work is the 12th century art of Hildegard of Bingen, entitled 'A *Study of Compassion. (Human) in Sapphire Blue*' (Plate 9).

What is *depicted* in the work of Hildegard of Bingen is the energy field surrounding the human form. What is *conveyed* is her ancient, and now contemporary, notion that the body resides in a field of consciousness, rather than consciousness residing in the body. In a book which contains this work of art, Matthew Fox (1985) points out that Hildegard spoke of the body/soul relationship in this imagery of a shared energy system, with the soul energy being the greater entity.

What is intriguing in this art is the fact that, at the aperture of the human form's head (as explained by Hildegard), 'this powerful healing energy can leave its own field and mix with others, and vice versa' (Fox 1985, p. 23). The sacred circle is also a feature of her work, conveying a similarity with certain traditions of tapestry, weaving and rituals that are common today among indigenous peoples around the world. This work captures symbolically the cosmic web of creation, the web of the universe, the interconnectivity of all being and of divinity with creation and humanity (Fox 1985, p. 23).

As a result of the ancient art and narrative of the 12th century Hildegard, combined with the contemporary art of the 20th century Alex Grey, combined with views from medical and social sciences, we see emerging views of the transpersonal body, human being and becoming, reinforced by notions of consciousness, unity, wholeness, energy and the connectedness of all, the sacred. Likewise, the premodern, modern, postmodern and beyond merge. They meet with a new spiraling of wisdom across time and space, and across all fields of inquiry and health practices. They invite us to reconsider our own being and becoming as health practitioners. The implications for the future are both ponderous and wondrous.

PLATE 1

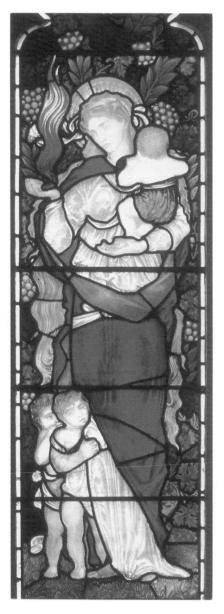

Plate 1 Return to core values: the timeless archetype of caritas nurse. ('Charity', detail from the window 'Faith, Hope and Charity' designed by Sir Edward Burne-Jones for Christ Church Cathedral. Oxford. © Woodmansterne Publications Ltd. Reproduced with permission.)

PLATE 2

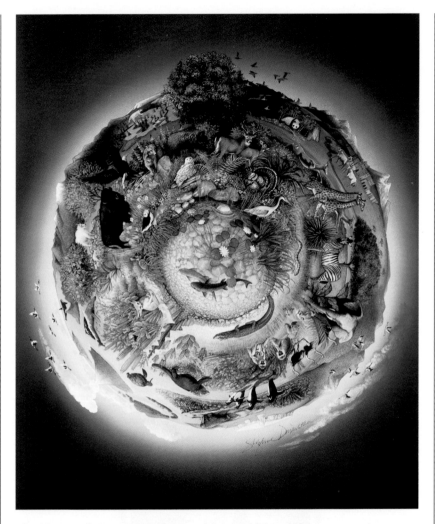

Plate 2 An artist's portrayal of the evolving worldview shift to an ecocaring cosmology, an inner and outer vision of wholeness and the connectedness of all life on earth. (© Suzanne Duranceau 1990. Reprinted with permission.)

PLATE 3

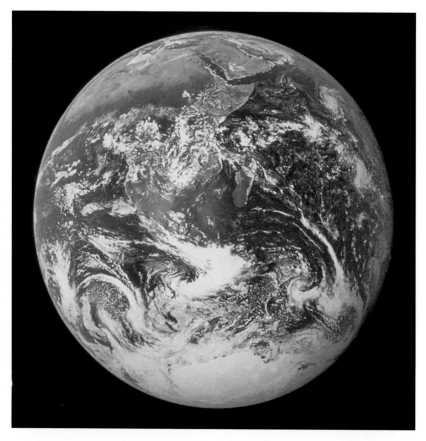

Plate 3 A caring cosmology evolves through concentric circles from self-other-nature-all living things to the furthest reaches of the universe, seeking the point of intersection between time and the timeless, the heaven and earth. (NASA Space Collection 'The Earth from Space'. Photo credit: NASA.)

PLATE 4

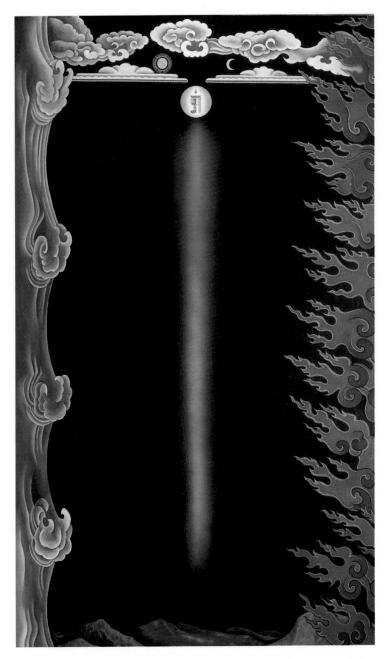

Plate 4 A depiction of the void/clear light consciousness as it arises out of the universal polar principles, symbolized here as the essence of opposing elements. (Void/Clear Light from *Sacred Mirrors* series by Alex Grey 1982. Reprinted with permission of Alex Grey.)

PLATE 5

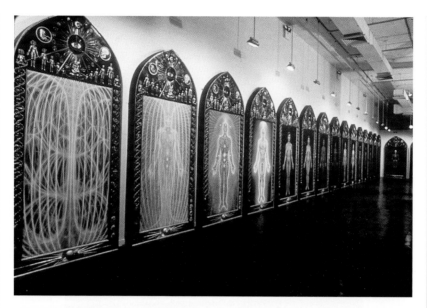

Plate 5 The 'Sacred Mirrors' sequence of paintings, showing views of the body from the physical to the metaphysical. (*Sacred Mirrors* series, installation view at New Museum, NYC, by Alex Grey 1986. Reprinted with permission of Alex Grey.)

PLATE 6

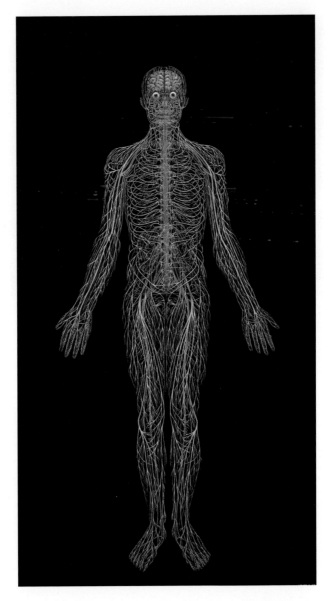

Plate 6 The nervous system from the 'Sacred Mirrors' series. (Nervous System from *Sacred Mirrors* series by Alex Grey 1979. Reprinted with permission of Alex Grey.)

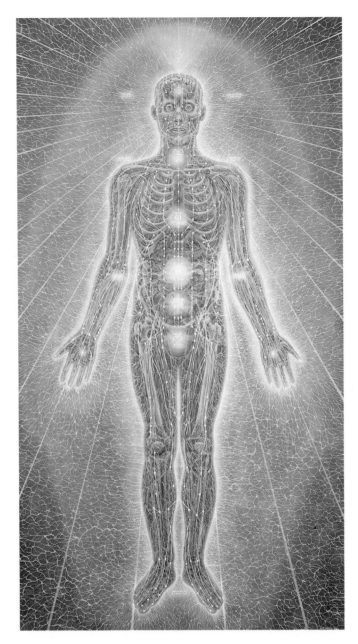

Plate 7A The yogic chakras and acupuncture meridians – the psychic energy system. (Psychic Energy System from *Sacred Mirrors* series by Alex Grey 1980. Reprinted with permission of Alex Grey.)

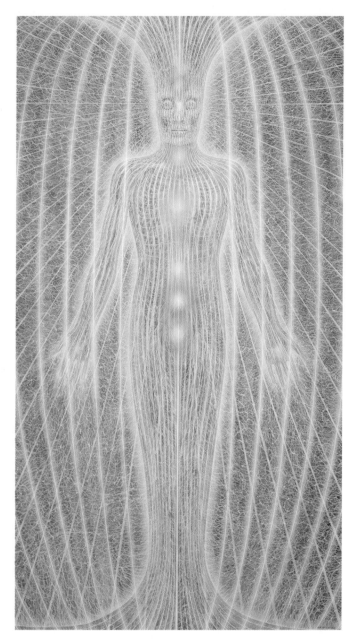

Plate 7B The yogic chakras and acupuncture meridians – the spiritual energy system. (Spiritual Energy System from *Sacred Mirrors* series by Alex Grey 1981. Reprinted with permission of Alex Grey.)

PLATE 8

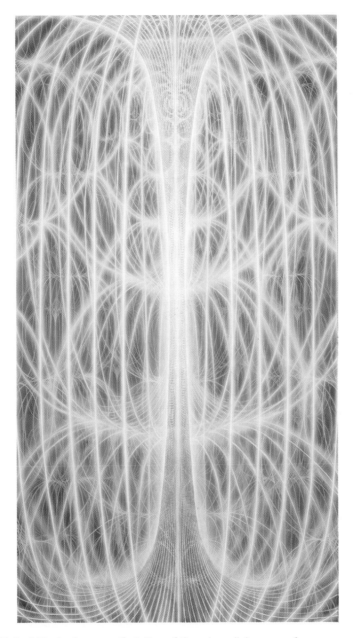

Plate 8 The body as manifestation of the primordial energy of awareness that is everywhere present. (Universal Mind Lattice from *Sacred Mirrors* series by Alex Grey 1981. Reprinted with permission of Alex Grey.)

PLATE 9

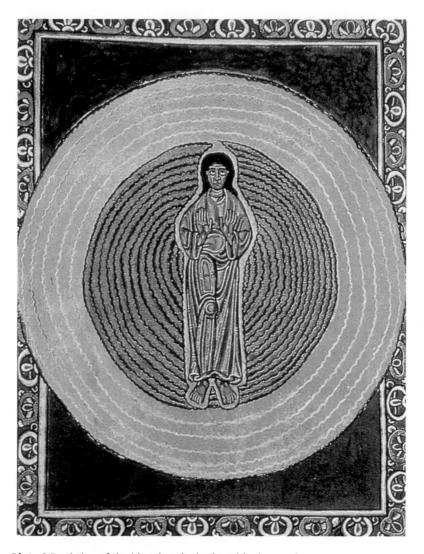

Plate 9 Depiction of the idea that the body resides in consciousness.
(From 'Illuminations of Hildegard of Bingen'. © Otto Müller Verlag, Salzburg 1954.
Reprinted with permission.)

12

Exercises for experiencing the transpersonal body

....

Love in all its subtleties is nothing more, and nothing less, than the more or less direct trace marked on the heart of the element by the psychical convergence of the universe upon itself. ...This is the ray of light which will help us to see more clearly around us.

(Teilhard de Chardin 1964, p. 265)

In entering into a transpersonal model for caring and healing, one starts with self. While there are numerous routes to mindful practices, there are some experiences and exercises that can assist in accessing one's transpersonal self.

Centering exercise

One approach I use is a basic quieting, centering exercise. One can either lie down or sit upright in a sitting position or with crossed legs in a lotus-type position. Begin by closing your eyes and becoming aware of your breath; breathe deeply, relaxed and easily. As you go inside yourself, find that quiet place that we all have access to. Go there and be still within yourself, even momentarily.

Once you are in that quiet, inner place, allow yourself to feel how good it is to be quiet and still. See if you can dwell there and feel the lovely sensation of just being still and quiet, accessing a sense of inner peace.

As you continue with the experience, allow yourself to breathe clearly and easily. As you continue to breathe, things will come to mind that take you beyond your breathing and quiet center; just observe the process, but return to that quiet space.

As you release your breath, gently release and let go of anything that comes into your mind, or anything that is bothering you, knowing that everything is changing. All of life is a process of expansion and contraction, and each breath brings new life and new light into you. Each exhalation allows you the opportunity to release and let go of anything that is bothering you. Each time return to that quiet place inside, dwell there, and remember how good it is to be still. You may stay in this place for 5 minutes or more.

When you are ready, return to your awake, alert state, feeling refreshed and cleared, cleansed in mind and body and more present to self, others and the present moment, and more available to life.

From this quiet centering as a beginning, the exercise can go in many directions: to mindful body meditation; focused visualization; concentrated meditation on the chakra systems; simple breath work; or to a range of meditative, contemplative practices, such as centering prayer, chanting, mantra meditations, and so on. The body exercise may be a useful one to continue with here.

Connecting with the body

To move forward from a quieting, centering experience to connecting with the body, simply lie down on your back and stretch out in a comfortable position on a mat or carpet. Feel yourself in your body; explore your body and gently note points of tension. Allow your attention to gently flow through your body and detect any feelings, positive or negative, that may be present in the various parts of the body.

Notice which parts of the body seem alive and strong, and which parts heavy, dull, tight, full, even painful. Without judging the feelings and sensations, just note them and continue to breathe, letting the feelings and attention flow easily.

You may find yourself wandering out of your body and becoming aware of where you are, if not in your body. When this happens, gently return to the breathing and the body awareness, noting the sensations and being present with them. If you find yourself being frustrated and impatient, note these thoughts and feelings as well, noting where they manifest in the body, and continue with the process. Do not give up until you feel a sense of peace and quiet that you can be present to. The thing we think of as being inside us—a self—actually is a personality, an ego and body sensation that rises and passes as part of an effortless flow of nature (Young 1994). As you work mindfully with this process, you realize that the deep, inner self, the transpersonal self, is actually more like 'no-self', and you can learn to let go of your ego self. One can cultivate the practice to the extent that one can have an inner sense of happiness, independent of circumstances.

You may continue with this process of being in your body for 15 minutes or more. If you have pain or tense sensations in any body area, observe the sensation as much as possible, with a sense of detached, but engaged, non-judgmental, accepting interest. You may send loving thoughts to different parts of the body, honoring the body experience and what it is needing to communicate to you.

Observe, breathe and release; continue gently and easily; being still in your body and honoring being present to self. Once you have explored the body and experienced the sensations, you can move to more focused breathing, concentrating on a given word, or a visual image that comforts and soothes you. You may chose to place yourself somewhere beautiful and safe; go there and nurture yourself, but remain focused within the experience, trying not to daydream at random. If that happens, return to focusing on your breathing and being in your body, or staying with the experience you want to create to nurture yourself. Remember to stay with the process, which will deepen with practice.

When you are ready you can return to a more whole-bodied, full-minded awareness of being.

When we can learn to witness our changing thoughts, emotions and inner-mind chatter, then we begin to realize that we are more than these passing thoughts, emotions and desires. If these passing experiences can be witnessed as rising and falling, expanding and contracting, then they no longer threaten in the same way as before.

Even if anxiety is present, we can catch ourselves 'in process', observing the moment, no longer being tied to the feeling or thought, no longer having to resist or run from it, knowing that this, too, is passing. As we learn to be a 'transpersonal witness' (Wilber 1981), we can simply watch these movements pass by and through us, leaving inner calm, serenity, and a sense of peace.

As one continues to cultivate a contemplative, meditative practice becoming still within and being present to the body and the deep, inner self, one increasingly becomes connected with the transpersonal dimension of life. As you continue to practice, you begin to experience personally how the ego mind and body awareness exercises and practices help you to change both, by realizing the oneness of all. The body-physical reaches down to earth to feel its density and ground of support, while also reaching upward to heaven to feel the light and space and inner wholeness of being (Wilber 1981). By cultivating one's own practice, opposites begin to dissolve and unite, and a deeper unity of all is discovered and experienced.

It is here that one can also practice conscious states of holding loving kindness, compassion and a caring consciousness toward self and others and the world. From this awareness and ongoing practice, one's subjective state and consciousness begin to translate into objective actions in the world, actions that bring loving, kindness and benefit to others.

Then, as one pursues the body practice, it becomes a spiritual awakening; as one pursues a spiritual practice, it is a transpersonal body awakening. One becomes the route to the other and vice versa. One begins to intuit a deep, inward sense of calm, serenity, freedom, lightness, relief and 'centeredness'. Even in the midst of hectic situations, one seeks to reside in that centered place, retaining calmness and stillness in the midst of raging anxiety and chaos among us.

Eventually, mind, body and soul are embodied in one moment of being. Life becomes a series of moments of being present. Being centered in each moment is one of the goals of life and practice within the transpersonal paradigm. As one awakens to the need to cultivate a contemplative, centering practice for self, then one becomes more aware of what might be meant by the concept of authentic presence, holding an intentional caring consciousness and a professional reflective practice. One then becomes more aware of the need for ongoing spiritual, ontological development, if one is to engage in caring–healing work.

This pursuit of spiritual practice then becomes the ground of our being, and the ground of any professional caring–healing practices. This returns health professionals to a deep commitment to service, to following one's talents and gifts, practicing from an authentic ethic of one's own being.

In considering this model, one then becomes aware that the transpersonal dimension is indeed an ontological view of life and practice. The model assists us in evolving beyond the horizontal, circling path that keeps us confined to the physical–material plane of existence. This professional and personal path is both immanent and transcendent, allowing for conscious choice, spiritual growth and ontological development. In cultivating one's transpersonal self, one experiences the 'at-one-ment' of all. May you be graced on your spiritual journey and deepened through your contemplative practices, whatever they may be.

> It is only by making ... moral experiments that we can discover the intimate nature of mind and its potentialities. In the ordinary circumstance of average sensual life, these potentialities of the mind remain latent and unmanifest.

> (Harman 1987b)

13

Professional ontological competencies for transpersonal practice

....

What about a model that inspires? That shows us what we would like to become, and infuses us with the ideas and strength needed to approximate it.

(Smith 1982)

Within this paradigm, the next phase of evolution leads us to consider how these premises and assumptions related to the transpersonal dimensions of caring–healing can generate professionally cultivated ontological competencies for transpersonal caring–healing practices. The following competencies come to mind as a starting point. Some of these capabilities are already present among so-called healing practitioners, and are considered mainstream within the field of alternative medicine (Fig. 13.1). They include the following:

- Invocation of the sacred; cultivation of a sense of the reverent in caring and healing processes of life and existence in the universe.
- Realization that caring is ultimately an ontology—a way of being; it calls forth a practice whereby one 'shares one's energy of being' and holds an intentional consciousness toward self and others; i.e., the one caring holds higher-frequency thoughts and caring consciousness as primary; this higher frequency of caring consciousness in turn helps to soothe, or calm, or potentiate

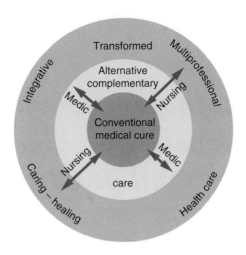

Figure 13.1 Evolving medical–health care approaches.

wholeness of a person with a lower-frequency system
(which is often the case if someone is ill, or suffering).

The model asks the professional to *be with* another on their journey of health and illness and healing.

When I first publicly suggested this idea of sharing one's energy, consciousness, or 'being' with another, I was criticized by some colleagues who said this thinking was not scientific enough. I have, nevertheless, pursued this line of thinking; it is also becoming more widely accepted as our paradigm of science shifts, and new explanatory models emerge.

I recently was heartened when I read Lamendola's (1994, in: Newman M 1994, p. 103) insight into his praxis, when he reported: 'I soon realized that all I had to do was "be there"...' In the same book, Newman also describes and discusses the notion of sharing consciousness as integral to the nurse–client relationship. She references her correspondence with Margi Martin in New Zealand, who wrote about the sharing of consciousness as part of the rhythmic coming together and moving apart that occurs in the nurse–client relationship.

Within this transpersonal model the following premises emerge:

- Caring as consciousness/consciousness as energy. Caring within a holographic perspective calls forth a need to be aware of, skilled in and willing to cultivate one's ability to ground, energize and center self and other. For example, within the transpersonal, Era III/Paradigm III consciousness, all caring, health and healing practitioners will need to know how to replenish energy, share energy and shift their field of consciousness.

- Caring as an ontology elicits the practitioner holding high-frequency energy thoughts such as love, caring, forgiveness and kindness. This awareness calls forth from the practitioner an awakening toward holding (or seeking to hold) and manifesting a caring–healing consciousness in each caring moment. This consciousness is enhanced with a focused intentionality to potentiate wholeness, harmony and healing.

- Caring–healing consciousness calls forth the concept and practice of 'being mindfully present'—holding compassion, equanimity and a non-judgmental stance.

- The need to cultivate the ability to be authentically present to self and other; to open to the experience of 'at-one-ment' within a single caring moment; attending to and connecting with the spirit condition of the other as part of the transpersonal experience.

- Consciousness as energy calls forth an awareness of one's state of consciousness and of how to cultivate the ability to be 'mindfully present'; to receive and release negative energy/consciousness; to foster how to direct caring–healing consciousness and energy to self and other. This awareness evokes the need for regular spiritual, contemplative, meditative centering practice from the practitioner.

- The regular practice of transpersonal self characteristics assists in cultivating competencies in connecting with self and other for subjective–intersubjective understanding; in acquiring meaning, and deeper understanding, beyond facts per se; in engaging in hearing and honoring one's personal story, narrative of meaning, sacred meanings and/or spiritual aspects of the soul journey towards healing.

- The relational spiritual aspect of caring–healing calls for the practitioner to connect with his or her higher/deeper self, for reflective/contemplative practices within a moral context; to open to a new science of unitary consciousness.

- A unitary consciousness foundation for transpersonal caring calls forth an openness to wonder, to mystery and to a sense of the sacred; a reverential perspective towards self, other, nature and the living cosmos. It involves cultivating an attitude of respect and awe of the unknown and undertaking new explorations to learn one's potential to access the inner healing processes.

- The transpersonal model requires an ability to convey authentic caring and the loving acceptance of other(s).

- It manifests intuitive, personal, aesthetic and ethical knowledge, skills and understanding.

- It requires an ability to engage and be responsive within a relationship of mutuality.

- It requires an ability to be vulnerable and connect with other(s) in meaningful, trusting relationships.

- The ontological–sacred consciousness dimensions of transpersonal caring–healing calls forth a commitment to ontological competencies and ontological development, i.e. a commitment to one's own personal practices.

- The transpersonal caring model incorporates soul care—fostering ongoing self-growth, spiritual growth and healing for the wounded healer.

As we begin to open to the postmodern and beyond framework, we begin to see nursing (and other) practices that are based upon an ontology of caring. We begin to see manifestations of a transpersonal orientation, even though it may not be named as such. The next section will help us consider the ontological competency shift in action, through exemplars.

Ontologically based nursing practices

In modern nursing, caring was reduced to 'care', as a noun, or as a verb. It was usually translated as caring for bodies and illness symptoms, or caring for machines and undertaking treatments, functional tasks and skills. Nursing in the modern context was manifested by an outward state of being, translated into nursing as *doing*. The way of 'doing caring' became a form of nursing/caring as technology; the nurse became a mechanic of sorts, or a deliverer of mechanical care.

Within the modern era of nursing, there was little attention to nurses' state of consciousness or ways of being. One's consciousness was not considered relevant to the nurse's ability to 'do care'; nurses were tied up being busy. However, as a colleague in England put it, 'being busy is a moral state' (Pyrce, personal communication 1994). Being busy is a *choice*.

In the shift from modern to an emerging postmodern/transpersonal consciousness, there is a shift from the horizontal path of doing, exemplified by 'caring as technology', to the vertical path of 'caring as an evolving ontology', discussed above. In this framework, the caring practitioner has to cultivate a caring consciousness as part of the healing process; this requires self-development and ongoing spiritual growth.

This shift has profound and dramatic consequences for nursing education and practices. There are indications that such practices are already present among us, or are emerging around the world.

International/national nursing examples of ontologically based caring practices and scholarship

Examples are already evident in nursing models that attend to an ontology of being as part of the foundation for nursing education, scholarship and health care practices. This section highlights some of the activities in which I have been personally involved, and which will hopefully serve as inspirations to others.

For example, nurses in Portugal have instituted a nursing clinical orientation that makes their ontological orientation explicit for the persons they serve. Maria de Fatima Rosado Marques and Manuel Lopes at the Hospital Distrital de Evona, and an adjoining nursing school, Escola de Enfermagen de Sao Joaode Deus in Lisbon, have a new clinical program that reveals the ontological orientation. Their literature states the following:

> People who come to us come in a free and spontaneous way, and are with us as long as they wish. We offer:

- An unconditional response, free from criticism and judgment.
- A space of freedom, solidarity and human authenticity.
- An empathic understanding.
- A positive listening.   (Marques & Lopes, personal communication, 1994)

This Portuguese example is consistent with the transpersonal caring ontology explicated above. The caring ethic is evident, as is the authenticity of being, a critical aspect of a caring ontology. The nurses make the non-judgmental aspect of the relationship explicit. There are increasing examples of an ontological orientation emerging in nursing centers and projects in different parts of the USA and other parts of the world. While those in the samples may not define their orientation as ontological or even transpersonal, the examples nevertheless have such components.

An illustration of a caring ontology and the importance of the 'being' of the professionals is evident in some of the guidelines put forth by the National Health Service (NHS) in the UK in its 1992 Health Report (DOH). The guidelines include the following:

1. That the relationship between (patient) and ... caregivers is recognized as being of fundamental importance.
2. That schemes should be set up enabling (patients) to get to *know one or two health professionals* ... who will *be with them* during their (needs) ... whether at home or in hospital, and who will continue the care ... [author's italicization].

Again, these guidelines imply and make explicit the importance of ontological competencies for transpersonal caring or relationship-centered care. The emphasis is on *relationship, being with, constancy* and *continuity*, concepts that are fundamental to a caring ontology and awareness, regardless of the nature of the illness, care needs, or technological demands the care requires.

In St Paul, Minnesota, nurses run a 'block nurse' program to provide coordinated services to elderly people to allow them to remain in their homes and receive convenient and appropriate high-quality care. Other examples occurring throughout the USA include some 120 000 nurses who have advanced education to practice nursing, freeing them to practice nursing qua nursing, without the traditional modern, medical constraints or ideology (American Nurses Association 1995).

Newman (1994) has also reported on several exemplary models of what I call ontologically based practices, which include a more integrative level of nursing, requiring a postgraduate level of education, and encompassing complex levels of care and pattern recognition, involving a partnership in a collaborative caring relationship. Examples include the 'Healing Web' project at the University of South Dakota and Augustana College (Koerner & Bunkers 1994, pp. 51–63), and the Carondelet St Mary's Health Center in Tucson. These nursing models emanate from a philosophical/theoretical base consistent with the unitary, transformative paradigm (Newman 1994, p. 129).

The activities at the Winter Haven Hospital in Florida, headed by Judy Cottrill and Libby Merle, represent another pocket of ontologically based clinical work, as does the Englewood Hospital in New Jersey. Both are recent experiments dedicated to caring-theory-based nursing practice. Both systems are facilitating nursing and nurses in developing advanced caring–healing practices and new models of care delivery, both in and outside the institution. Part of the effort encompasses, as it must, major professional development, educational programs and experiential learning opportunities.

The ontology of relationship characterized by compassion, continuity, respect for choice, unconditional acceptance and mutuality of growth, for both nurse and client, are all part of these national exemplars (Newman 1994, p. 129). They reflect new models of nursing practice which are grounded in caring, relationship and consciousness as the ontological basis for practice.

The recent work at Queens Medical Center in Honolulu, headed by the late Duane Walker, serves as another example of ontological shift thinking. The entire hospital, as I understand it, has undergone a major rethink of lits core values and commitment to native Hawaiian customs and healing beliefs, and has shifted to a focus on inner healing and the healing arts which honor the unity of mindbodyspirit. They have instituted professional development with ontologically based programs for staff and ultimately for patients. (They found they had to offer the experiences to staff before they could be authentically offered to patients.) These programs include classes and experiences in, for example, Tai Chi, meditation and massage.

The Queen' s nursing staff is also engaged in formal research programs related to, for example, therapeutic touch and other healing modalities, offered before and after surgery, with an examination of patient outcomes.

The North Hawaii Community Hospital project on the Big Island of Hawaii stands as another exemplar, helping to lead the way to a new world of health care. Under the leadership, devotion, commitment and undying efforts of Earl Bakken and the grass roots community of Hawaii, the 'hospital for the 21st century' has been born. Here, they offer the conventional Western model of care, augmented by traditional, native Hawaiian healers and complementary caring–healing practices such as healing touch. With the combined executive ability of Pat Linton, the Chief Executive Officer, and the clinical experience and philosophy of Jae Termeer, the Nursing Head, new innovations of caring–healing practices are occurring, within a transpersonal paradigm.

A project at The Children's Hospital in Denver, Colorado, which is connected with some of the work at the University of Colorado Center for Human Caring, is similarly focused. One of the critical oncology units, the HOT unit (hematology, oncology and transplant care), under the direction of Mary Jo Cleveland and associates Dr Jan Nyberg and Dr Phyllis Updike are conducting a social action research project. This clinical research project involves a formal program of staff development related to caring theory–philosophically guided practice.

The caring theory and philosophy are combined with opportunities for nurses to gain advanced clinical skills in a selected caring–healing modality. These modalities include healing arts such as therapeutic touch, music, massage and visualization. Placed within an ontological trans-personal paradigm, the modalities are integrated into conventional clinical nursing practice skills.

Other exemplars include some of the clinical scholarship and caring theory-based and theory-guided practice developments in Canada. The early work of Eileen Cappell (now Fitzpatrick) in the late 1980s and early 1990s, and the more recent work of Mary Jane McGraw and others in the Ontario area (and to some extent in Quebec and Montreal, such as Therese Doucet, Dr Chantal Cara and the early work of the late Dr Georgette Desjean) stand out as exemplars for transforming practice. The early collaborative project work of Dr Marcia Hills at Victoria University, British Columbia, with her colleagues in education throughout the province, has also provided new paradigm thinking and new educational models that represent the ontological shift proposed in this book.

More recently, a consortium of Canadian educators, administrators and clinicians is emerging within the Canadian system, and is working towards new paradigm thinking within the transpersonal caring model, seeking new system reforms. Canadian nursing has moved more quickly toward theory-based and theory-guided nursing practice than has its USA counterpart, leading to exciting leadership developments and experimentation.

I might mention as an aside that, directly or indirectly, one of the benefits of nursing theory and theory-guided practice (and reflective practice-guided theory) is that it helps clinicians and scholars alike to return to considering the ontological foundation of their practice. This ontological view assists in examining and critiquing basic values and paradigm premises about how one views person, humanity, environment, relationship, caring–healing, health and illness, suffering and wholeness. It helps one to examine and re-examine the role and purpose of nursing.

When these matters are seriously pursued, they help practitioners to reflect upon the ethics and philosophy behind their worldview and behind their actions. In doing so, transformation can result, from inside out. Theory-based nursing and health care are consistent with an ontological shift and movement toward the transpersonal model for the future. Use of appropriate theory is one way to move forward, assuming the theories are consistent with an open, emerging paradigm.

International examples of the ontological shift in nursing education and practice

Examples that are both nursing theory based and also ontologically oriented within a caring model include the works of Dr Katie Eriksson at Abo Akademi, Swedish University in Vasa, Finland, and also in Helsinki, Finland. There, in 1986, Dr Eriksson established the first Department of Caring Science. To my knowledge, this was the first academic department of its kind in the world. In 1992, this same department was designated as a distinct Faculty of Caring and Social Science.

As an academic department of caring science, its focus is on 'caritative' caring, based on a 'caritas motive' (that is, related to human love, hope and a caring society). This university academic department is based upon a foundational ontology of caring as a starting point and context for its epistemic and ontological studies and practices.

In Sweden, departments of nursing are housed in 'colleges of caring science' and university-based nursing and related health programs are referred to as 'caring sciences'. Although the Swedish developments are more recent than the Finnish developments in this area, the Swedish universities are also beginning to focus on the ontological and epistemic dimensions of caring.

Göteborg University in Sweden, under the early leadership of Professor Britt Johannson and educator Ference Marton, is advanced with respect to nursing pedagogy and advanced nursing education. Increasingly, its work is being developed within the caring science context. Norway is another country which has made the ontological focus of nursing science prevalent. Some Norwegian scholars are raising new questions about the philosophy of science in general, and about nursing and caring science in particular, for example: 'Can nursing–caring be a science? Or is it something that can only be studied at the ontological, ethical and philosophical level?' These are rhetorical questions for postmodern nursing.

The developments in the South Pacific, especially in Australia and New Zealand, are also occurring within an ontological context. Here, the focus is more on critical social theory and critiques of science and modern practices. They are seeking to uncover the hegemony of dominant medical ideologies and practices with conscious intentionality. In Australia, Professors Alan Pearson and Judy Lumby, Judith Parker, Annette Street, Jill White, Dot Angel and others, like Margi Martin and Alison Dixon in New Zealand, come to mind. Much of their scholarship and clinical models are emancipatory, designed as reflective, critical transformative models, whereby both individual and system practices are liberated, making caring–healing more possible.

Other efforts are prominent in the UK with the reflective practice work led by Christopher Johns and the work of Carole Cox at the City University in London, where her graduate programs and research are related to healing and advanced caring practices. The avant-garde work of Steve Wright, Jean Sayre-Adams, and Francis and Anna Biley are also examples of caring–healing work representing the ontological level preparation. In the Scottish Highlands, Dr Betty Farmer has an on-going community–academic vision for integrating models of caring into social programs.

Developments are occurring in Thailand and, to some extent, in Japan. These countries are recognizing the relationship between their cultural traditions of contemplative, Zen-mindfulness practices, and the trans-personal model of caring and healing. This awakening is providing more confidence and more freedom for nurse educators and scholars to return to some of the ancient knowledge and wisdom of their cultures. For example, the practice of meditation and of attending to a 'caring moment' (being 'mindfully present' and 'authentically available') are inherent to the contemplative meditative practices of their people. They are learning how to reincorporate this basic ontological work into their individual and system changes and into their educational and clinical scholarship and models for practice.

Some similar activities are occurring among nursing scholars and leaders in South America. Alcione Laite de la Silva, Eloita Neves Arruda and their Brazilian colleagues are working to develop a transformative-transcendent paradigm for nursing education and practice in Brazil. Such work is generating a critical mass of informed and dedicated nursing leaders and interdisciplinary health colleagues, working together to create new healing models for a new millennium.

All of these national and international nursing leaders and their post-modern works are aimed at ushering in a new paradigm for the next century. All of these exemplars reside within a transpersonal model, or are moving toward the transpersonal, even though the work may not have been labeled as such.

The University of Colorado Center for Human Caring

The last example of activities at the ontological level of development is the University of Colorado Center for Human Caring, which I established in 1986, as the first of its kind. The Center for Human Caring was originally designed to be an 'experimental think tank' for the School of Nursing. Its work has the philosophical–ontological–epistemological level as its foundation.

The Center's focus has been on exploring new ways to advance the art and science of human caring. These efforts have ranged from specific curricular activities to new educational-researched practice models. The Center encourages special initiatives that foster some of the epistemo-logical, ontological, methodological and praxis inquiries associated with new ways of knowing and thinking and being in a caring relationship. Some of the published information about the center includes the following (Watson 1992a):

> Formal faculty associates in the Center are exploring such areas as the moral and
> philosophical basis of caring, caring ethics, the role of humanities in a caring
> curriculum, and the teaching and practice of caring.

The Center also fosters nontraditional, contextual, methodological investigations through approaches such as hermeneutics, phenomenology, literary analysis, and writing/narrative as method. Traditional empirical pursuits or methodological combinations are also fostered, in addition to methods that explore the 'shared humanness' of caring and healing and the ontological interconnections between humans, between humans and nature, and between the one-caring and the one-cared-for.

Consistent with the nature of caring knowledge, the Center for Human Caring advocates an interdisciplinary approach to the study and teaching of human caring; it draws directly upon the underdeveloped connections between humanities, human caring and healing practices, while not neglecting traditional biomedical knowledge and practices. Collaborative programs between and among other academic units on the Health Sciences Center and other campuses in the university are ongoing.

Some of the outcomes of the Colorado Center include the international demonstration project called 'The Denver Nursing Project in Human Caring', which is a nursing-managed center for persons who are human immunodeficiency virus (HIV) positive or living with acquired immuno-deficiency syndrome (AIDS). This project, from its origins in 1988 to 1996, became an exemplar of a model reflecting caring at all levels in its programs, activities and clinical and administrative practices. Nursing colleagues from around the world have visited the Denver Nursing Project to experience the ontological level of the caring theory in action. Early project directors such as Dr Janet Smerke and, later, Dr Ruth Neil have served as hosts to hundreds of professional visitors. Some of the publications from the project continue to influence clinical initiatives and serve as theory-led practice guidelines for non-conventional medical and health care.

Whole-person-centered caring was offered to clients and others who referred themselves to the project. The care modalities ranged from basic medical treatments, respiratory care and blood work, to nutrition educational counseling, a range of touch modalities, exercise physiology programs, client-centered work programs, and a caring partnership model of managed care. Although the project is no longer running, the model continues to inspire similar models elsewhere.

During the early to mid 90s, international affiliate activities of the Center emerged in other parts of the world. They include sites in the Scottish Highlands in the UK; The Baycrest Gerontology Center in Ontario, Canada; the Collaborative Nursing Education Project in Victoria, British Columbia, Canada; and Victoria University Department of Graduate Nursing in Wellington, New Zealand. As these affiliate activities have emerged and changed, they have been augmented by an emerging network of national and international colleagues who are generating new consortia models. The Center is engaged in collaborative, consultative programs and collegial relationships with colleagues in hospitals and clinical and academic settings in other sites around the world. In addition to those already mentioned, these include Taiwan, Korea, Germany and Micronesia. The latest developments are formally merging Center activities into an international Center concept for the University of Colorado School of Nursing (1998).

All of the institutions and individuals involved in networks with the Center for Human Caring are engaged in study, practice and educational and research programs and projects that adhere to caring as an ontology. Caring is viewed as an ontology, as ethic, as ethos, and as a central epistemic and clinical focus, essential to the mature development of the discipline of nursing.

In addition, there are nursing theory-guided activities which are increasing around the USA and other parts of the world. Whenever nursing and nurses begin to develop reflective practice models that are guided by a philosophical and theoretical nursing perspective, they almost invariably incorporate caring as an ontology, even if they do so without naming it as such.

The postmodern–transpersonal Era II/Paradigm III model presented here for caring–healing acknowledges, and is informed by, numerous other advances in nursing and health care generally. But this model, while building upon extant work in nursing and related fields in the USA and other parts of the world, goes beyond 'what is', while also incorporating 'what is already inscribed' in nursing worldwide, 'on the margins'.

While the international examples given here reflect some of the most exciting contemporary efforts to advance nursing as the art and science of human caring, within an ontological foundation, they also reflect the paradigm shift that is already emerging around the world. There is already inscribed, on the margin, a movement within nursing away from an exclusive focus on 'modern technological competencies' to 'the ontological competencies' necessary for a transpersonal caring–healing paradigm.

My work is but one of many attempts to locate that promising marginal text (ontology of caring) and to disclose it using a different lens, so that we might see it in a new light. Then it can be more fully developed, rather than subsumed, assumed, taken for granted, or excluded altogether (which is what seemed to happen during the modern Era I/Paradigm I and, to some extent although less so, during Era II/Paradigm II).

In order for nursing to mature into its own postmodern paradigm, it must move, once again, towards the paradox of being beyond nursing. Consistent with the phenomena of caring and the human health/healing experiences, we need to make explicit the professional 'ontological competencies' expected for the advancement of nursing, and all health care practitioners' transpersonal caring–healing practice. As we openly acknowledge the ontological shift, and that 'competencies of being' are essential for transpersonal care, we naturally begin to attend to the artistry of healing work. Then we see the connection between ontological competencies and the way in which they can be translated into professional caring–healing modalities.

The next section considers the healing arts as manifestations of ontological competencies. We can also see how they can be integrated into conventional medicine, while acknowledging that they are essential for transpersonal caring and healing practices.

Healing arts and the nurse/healing practitioner

Beauty and art

Beauty and art are part of the ushering in of a transpersonal caring–healing perspective. All true works of healing are works of beauty; beauty heals. In Emerson's words:

> *This element (beauty) I call an ultimate end. No reason can be asked or given why the soul seeks beauty. Beauty, in its largest and profoundest self, is one expression of the universe.*   (Emerson 1982, p. 48)

The Native American people remind us that 'every day we should do an act of power and an act of beauty.' Matthew Fox (1991) says we should shower one another with beauty, for as we do so, we bring out the beauty of one another. Others say one of the main obligations in life is to be as beautiful as we can in every way. Rumi, the ancient poet, posed that we let the beauty that we are, be what we do. In this way of thinking about art and beauty, every caring act becomes a potential act of beauty, and thus an act of healing.

Gablik (1991) identified two traditions in the modern art world:

- 'Artlike art', separate from life and everything else
- 'Lifelike art', art that is connected to life and to everything else.

Gadamer (1986) asserted that, by understanding art as a realm divorced from everyday life, aesthetics come to be viewed as separate from the truth. In his work, *The Relevance of the Beautiful*, he challenged the idea of art as a special, magical realm by pointing out the continuity between the world of art and our everyday world. He reminded us that we cannot encounter the work of art without being transformed in the process, in some way (Gadamer 1986, p. xiv). In reconsidering art, caring and healing, Gadamer allows us to view art as an experience of connection and continuity with the everyday world and therefore creates an opportunity for art to transform us.

Gablik (1991) framed the differences between modern and postmodern art by pointing out that when art and science are not cut off or uncoupled from the life world, they have characteristics which are resistant to institutional, capitalist and patriarchal imperatives, even though subsumed under them.

In educator and philosopher Maxine Greene's view (1991), it is the arts which move us into a space where we can create visions of other ways of being, and ask what it might signify to realize them. In health care, as in education, she notes:

> *I do not see how we can educate [heal] ... persons if we do not enable them on some level to open spaces for themselves—spaces for communicating across the boundaries, for choosing, for becoming different in the midst of intersubjective relationships.*   (Greene 1991, p. 28, author's parentheses)

It is in the engagement and re-engagement of the arts, in the art of being human, that humans will be less likely to confine themselves to the main text, to coincide forever with what they are. It is this quality of art which evokes images of liberation, which overcomes invisibility and that which has become 'normalized' (Greene 1991, p. 28). For it is the arts, and attending to a sense of beauty, which give rise to wonder, to questioning and to pondering our being.

The emergence of beauty and art into healing practices attaches to caring as an act of beauty, whereby the one-caring connects with and reflects the beauty of the soul to the one-cared-for, one to the other. Since our souls require beauty to be, how can we not honor beauty in our life, our caring practices, our institutions and our systems of healing?

Art is a way of dealing with life and healing processes in a reverential way, with a sense of awe and respect for the larger picture of the universe, leading to a moral shaping of our systems of healing. Where art is based upon 'caring for the whole and taking it to heart', it becomes more purposeful, challenging the dominant, modern medical paradigm by closing the gap between art, life and healing.

In this perspective, art is attuned to the laws of existence (McNiff 1992, p. 20). This is consistent with Kandinsky's view (1977) that the spiritual resides in art, and art bestows archetypal significance to the soul, for soul recovery. In McNiff's view, art 'ensouls' the world, invoking symbolic and varied aspects of our thoughts.

As an ontological shift emerges within society and models of health care, we see the public pursuing multiple approaches toward health and healing, calling forth this transpersonal caring context. We see attempts to reintegrate art and science in ways that are morally, socially, esthetically and ecologically grounded by being accountable to a larger whole; to healing self, other and Mother Earth. As Gablik (1991, p. 144) put it: 'Nothing which is not socially or ecologically responsible will make it out of this decade [the1990s] alive'.

New relationships are being established between art and healing. Within the transpersonal caring–healing perspective, we restore artistry and creativity to our practices and our lives. As we experience and enter into the artistic process of being and becoming, we literally and metaphorically become transformed. It is 'the pas de deux between art and life' (McNiff 1992, p. 38).

The healing arts are emerging from daily life and grassroots movements, showing us the healing potentials in visual arts, music, dance, theater, storytelling, design, architecture and other related areas. At least four types of healing arts have been identified that represent major approaches taken by contemporary artists engaged in healing arts. These categories are (Lafo, Capasso & Roberts 1994, p. 9):

- *Art intended to directly heal.* Such works use symbols or abstract images to promote wellness and to calm and center physical and spiritual responses. It includes works that activate specific physiological responses through positive visualization and soothing scenes. Alex Grey's 'Life energy system' and other works within the *Sacred Mirrors* series may be examples of this type of art (see Plates 7–10).

- *Art created by artists to facilitate their own personal healing.* This type of art is often autobiographical and involves highly charged abstract or representational body imagery. Examples of this type can be seen in women's art related to breast cancer. Other healing arts projects such as that in the Shane Hospital, University of Florida, Medical Arts program, fall within this category.

- *Art about aspects of the healing process.* These works of art reflect and comment on human experiences of healing and illness such as pain, loss, grief and body image changes, as well as hope, change and even spiritual transformations related to the complexities of healing. Some examples within this category include Edvard Munch's 'The Scream', and the Breast Cancer Women's Art Series (see below).

- *Artist-designed psychoarchitecture/healing space, healing architecture.* This use of art for healing makes a conscious, intentional effort to integrate symbol, myth, archetype, metaphor and mystery into architectural and environmental themes of healing, into health care facilities and new systems and healing models. This category captures some of the emerging notions related to recreating healing temples and returning to health-spa models that consciously attend to 'ontological design'. It includes, for example, the reintegration of sacred architecture into health care structures and systems, so humans can 'be' in a different way, experiencing self and the environment as a healing space (see Figure 16.4, p. 251). New structures are being developed in different parts of the world, such as Scandinavia, Hawaii and parts of Europe, where there is an

> attempt to consciously and intentionally use light, color, shape,
> form, lines, curves and nature for their ability to directly heal and/or
> to facilitate personal (or community) healing.

The conscious attention to art and all its many forms and uses is based on the ontological assumption that art is *life affirming*. Art touches and stimulates deep psychic healing energies at the archetypal level of consciousness. The creativity of the healing energy of art is a counterpoint to degeneration and disintegration. Art has power—not just the power of metaphor, symbol, myth, and self-expression—but a real operant power that can affect transformations, change lives and truly heal (Lafoo, Capasso & Roberts 1994).

Art that heals in all its dimensions accesses the human soul—the life force and archetypeal healing energy that lies dormant in each human being.

McNiff (1992) writes about the shamanic cultures worldwide which describe illness as a loss of soul. The shaman's task is to go on a journey in search of the abducted or lost soul and return it to the sick person (p. 19). Within the transpersonal, art and artistry at all levels play a much more conscious, intentional and prominent role. This ranges from the caring–healing modalities of art expression to healing art space that allows us to participate in a deep experience of humanity, shared across time. This care of the soul is increasingly being reintegrated into conventional and non-conventional practices. The arts help patients and practitioners to remember our soul and our deep longings for life-affirming messages. These messages remind us and reconnect us to a source of personal and collective empowerment (McNiff 1992, p. 19).

Art work as a work of creation has therapeutic–healing value, both for viewing as well as a form of expression. Healing images and archetypal visions emerge from such art healing. For example, in the area of women and breast cancer, a famous work by Chistiane Corbats, 'Amazon Cry for

Life', is a one-breasted armor-plated figure. The work says 'I am Amazon warrior' (Lafo, Capasso & Roberts 1994, p. 19).

Another example of art and breast cancer is Nancy Fried's work of sculpture, which reveals a woman who has had a mastectomy. The work mirrors and reflects back to us the shared recognition of anguish, loss, suffering, mutilation of body and person, yet personal strength and recovery—all in one art work.

Yet another example of the role of art is captured by a cancer patient who brought paintings, music, shells and photographs to her hospital room, attempting to create her own environment for healing. She described how the benefits exceeded her initial intention:

> Before I began bringing my living room to the hospital with me, I was just another disease. Nurses would often come into the room and never even make eye-contact with me. After I brought in the artwork and music, they began to notice the paintings, and ask me questions about the music. I became a person to them instead of just another illness. (McNiff 1992, p. 18)

Such examples point out that art actually serves to humanize and revitalize health care for both patient and practitioner. Such healing art connects us with our deepest self, our soul, as well as with our common humanity—the universal soul. Such healing art also both mirrors and makes visible our collective suffering and inner healing journey toward soul and toward wholeness.

Understanding the transpersonal model helps us to emphasize the importance of including arts in the design of healing spaces, as well as incorporating art into the daily environment. The rapid growth of art and healing architecture into hospitals and clinical programs is another example of the shift from *technologically designed* hospitals for the treatment of disease, to *ontologically designed* clinical systems (healing centers) geared toward art, beauty and expressive modalities as a therapeutic healing approach. Such an approach attends to the 'ills of the soul and the psyche', as well as to the body-physical treatment concerns which were dominant in the 'modern' design and treatment systems.

This new/old thinking acknowledges the therapeutic value and the process of expression and creation for healing mind, body and soul as one. We see more clearly that during the 19th century we moved from spa models to 'pest houses'—early treatment institutions or 'poor houses' where people were abandoned and mistreated, houses infested by pests, with a lack of sanitation, etc. These had to be reformed at the turn of the 20th century to produce modern, highly functional, disconnected, sterile, institutional settings. For the 21st century, we return to an integrated approach to health care. (This subject is discussed more fully in Chapter 16.)

Ultimately, the power of art within the healing process lies in its ability to connect us with ourselves. As we reframe our views of art and science and reintegrate moral and compassionate acts of art as caring–healing acts, we might be awakening and breaking the bounds on the disenchanted and disenchantment with the modern models of art, science, caring and healing (Gablik 1991). As we once again see the significance of art in any healing journey:

> We are brought back from our lost soul wanderings into the map of clarity.
> We are brought back into the fullness of the picture, and into the fullness of our
> own lives. We are no longer lost and alone. We have found some new charts to
> guide us homeward.   (McNiff 1992, p. 20)

In transpersonal caring and healing, we will need to create and sustain the existence of a community of healers which is committed to the domain of art, beauty and soul care to accompany and transform the usual ways of doing medicine. Medicine itself will also have to be emancipated and transformed in the process. Each practitioner, each healing artist, so to speak, will need to reach towards the making of a common world whereby human, environmental and world healing and peace are the common goals.

The alternative to not re-engaging with beauty and arts, at whatever level, is to conform to the automatism of the main text, never glimpsing the wonder, wholeness or healing that lies, already, always inscribed in the margin of our hearts and the open universe. The arts and beauty allow us to imagine another way, a better way, another possibility of how things are, but also of how they might be.

14

Reconsidering Nightingale: professional ontological competencies as advanced caring–healing arts

Over-emphasis on technology tends to overshadow therapeutic modalities that can have real significance. Nurses must recognize that they do not create change in people, rather they participate in the process of change to the extent that they bring knowledge to the situation and recognize that the healing process has the potential for healing beyond that which we recognize today.

(Rogers 1992, p. 61)

From Nightingale's 1859 (1992 commemorative edition) *Notes on Nursing* we can reconsider advanced caring–healing arts as being integral to transpersonal practice. There are underpinnings in Nightingale's work which foreshadow nursing and health within a postmodern 21st century paradigm. In her vision of health, well nursing and sick nursing, she foresaw the need for fewer hospitals and the need for a differentiation of nursing for diverse areas of practice. She strongly advocated education and the use of science and statistical evidence, logic and intellect, together with passion and vision. She highlighted and outlined environmental, institutional and human care essentials that are now being rediscovered.

Nightingale emphasized the distinct nature of the knowledge base needed by nurses. She asserted that nurses and nursing could assist in the development of a healthy society. With respect to postmodern, trans-personal practices, Nightingale has provided a timeless blueprint for the 21st century. According to her views, there is a covenant relationship from nurse to patient, and from nurse to God; body and soul for both nurse and patient are as one (Bradshaw 1996). 'Nursing is a spiritual service, the care of the soul can never be separated from the care of the body' (Pearce 1969, p. 79, in: Bradshaw, 1996: 22).

With her prophetic vision of health and basic care essentials as a body–soul connection, we can reconsider the importance of caring–healing/nursing arts as non-invasive, non-intrusive, natural healing modalities. Today, they relate to soul care. As Macrae (1995) suggested, some of today's contemporary spiritual practices can be integrated into nursing education and practice. Such approaches are consistent with Nightingale's philosophy of linking the ego personality with the inward, spiritual consciousness. Practices such as yoga, meditation, imagery and related contemplative practices can therefore be used in a variety of settings. Rogers pointed out that Nightingale's proposal for nursing practice during her age was not so different from today's emerging caring–healing modalities. As Rogers suggested 'in today's language these include meditation, therapeutic touch, imagery, humor, and various other modalities, many of which are yet to come' (Rogers 1992, p. 60).

Within the context of this book, we can see how the caring–healing arts become extensions of ontological competencies. The two areas intersect as we consider a contemporary perspective on transpersonal caring–healing modalities.

Nightingale gave special attention to the significance of the environment and its relationship to healing. We are all familiar with her famous phase: 'put the patient in the best condition for nature to act upon him (sic)' (1992 commemorative edition, p. 75). Her focus was on the basics—clean air, light, proper nutrition and sanitation. She also empha-sized variety: a view of the outdoors, a change in surroundings, paintings, color, flowers, plants and music. She mentioned spending time with pets and the role of children and infants in 'speeding recovery' (1992 commemorative edition).

Within Nightingale's model and within a postmodern/transpersonal cosmology, the areas she identified for 'health', can be translated into essential, caring–healing modalities comprising the finest of nursing arts— 'essentials' for knowledgeable caring practices. As Rogers framed it: 'The answer to health will not be found in more drugs, more technology, or more hospitals' (p. 61). The answer to health resides in a different framework than that of conventional medical treatment models. We are just beginning to comprehend the profound differences, the transformative thinking, required to fully consider health and healing.

Nightingale's metaparadigm focused on people and their world as the uniqueness of nursing, consistent with the latest thinking in nursing science. Nightingale's nursing was embedded in a continually changing evolutionary process, also consistent with emerging Era III/Paradigm III thinking of this time, of 'new visions, including energy fields, wave phenomena, and even space potentials' (1992 commemorative edition), all of which have new meaning within postmodern/transpersonal thinking. Postmodern reconsiderations of Nightingale provide a foundation for the emergence of a new world—a worldview and cosmology that unites earlier ideas with futuristic directions and new visions.

Some aspects of these visions were and are now basically spiritual. As Macrae (1995, p. 10) pointed out, following Nightingale's line of thought, we can help our patients clarify:

- 'the most valuable qualities they can bring forth from within
- the circumstances that are most helpful for the unfolding of these qualities
- ways of bringing about the circumstances or best conditions into their lifestyles'.

Part of this new vision includes uniting earlier ideas with those of the present and future with respect to basic and advanced caring–healing modalities.[1]

In addition to these modalities being extensions of my earlier work on the 'art of transpersonal caring' and on the 'carative factors', this perspective is also consistent with Newman's (1994, p. 112) description of the nurse–client relationship, in which there is a 'forming of shared consciousness (the interpenetration of the two fields)' as part of the process. Newman quoted Martin (1994, p.112), who identified 'attending to the explications (words, colors, skin, muscles, breathing, messages, images, spirit) of the client as explicit to the professional relationship and process of care'. This perspective is consistent with my discussion of the art of transpersonal caring, including 'scientific, artistic, humanistic, ethical and technical complexities, along with the emotional, mental, aesthetic, intuitive, physical, spiritual and experiential dimensions; that transpersonal nursing arts include "movement, touch, sounds, words, color, and forms" to transmit human to human transpersonal caring' (Watson 1988b, pp. 66, 68).

Finally, the so-called caring–healing modalities reconstructed here are informed by reconsidering Nightingale's timeless treatise and testimony about nursing. All of Nightingale's ideas, combined with some of the above work, are embedded 'on the margin' of modern nursing and emerging healing practices, waiting to be actualized for another century.

---

[1]In addition to Nightingale per se, the framing of these modalities under the physical sense organs was influenced by my colleague Dr Phyllis Updike in some of my discussions with her about new models for nursing. These areas are consistent to some extent with the sensory/perceptual category in the work on nursing diagnoses (even though I am not an advocate for 'nursing diagnosis' as such), by Kim, McFarland & McLane (1991, p. 55).

The notion of 'ontological competencies' was influenced by a speaker at a conference on 'Applied Heidegger' (University of California, Berkeley 1989), who spoke about 'ontological design' for computer programming. These modalities are extensions of my earlier work on 'carative factors' (Watson1979, reprinted 1985), and of my discussion below of the art of transpersonal caring (Watson 1988b, p. 66). My earlier work acknowledged nursing caring art as including 'movements, touch, sounds, words, colors, and forms' to transmit the art of caring (Watson 1988b, p. 68).]

Keep in mind that all of these reconstructed modalities are based upon a caring consciousness and intentionality to potentiate wholeness, harmony, integrity and beauty, and to preserve dignity and humanity with every act. These modalities are also comfort measures which serve to control pain, manage symptoms, soothe and relax, and to help create a sense of well-being through which natural healing can occur and the natural reparative processes can be facilitated.

The following sections are not intended to be comprehensive with respect to each modality. They are included to serve as a conceptual frame of reference in which to reconsider Nightingale's view of nursing arts, and the roots and relevance of her thinking today. Both the premodern and postmodern points of reference suggest that we have to reconsider the importance of caring arts for new reasons. In addition, both Nightingale and contemporary perspectives take on new meanings and new purposes for transpersonal caring–healing practices.

The following modalities 'from the margin', reframed, can become central transpersonal modalities. They are offered only as unfinished examples, with unlimited possibilities for expansion.

We see how Nightingale's premodern modalities were left under-developed and unattended to in the modern world of nursing and health care, but now are being reconsidered as fundamental to transpersonal caring and healing. It is important to see the roots of these new approaches that are emerging in nursing and other healing professions. They already exist 'on the margins' and can be found in Nightingale's original work, even though there is not a conscious awareness of the origins. Seen again, they carry a power and significance of their own, returning us to the most fundamental of nursing's caring arts, while advancing a mature post-modern/transpersonal practice. These nursing arts, reconsidered, span from Nightingale's premodern thinking through postmodern thinking, and incorporate the spiritual as well as the unity of physical care, emerging as transpersonal caring–healing modalities.

Transpersonal caring–healing modalities

Intentional, conscious use of auditory modalities

Premodern Nightingale caring arts 'from the margin'

The use of music and sound in healing is as old as humankind. The ancient healers drew upon our sense of sound and soundness for health and harmony, from Aesculapius to Socrates, Apollo, St Cecilia, and Hildegard of Bingen. The emerging physician, according to Don Campbell, will be the doctor of balance, fullness and resonance, relying upon a new understanding of the physics of harmonics and the powers of sound. In the 21st century, we will be able to 'use the beauty of musical sound to compose ourselves into a perfect octave of harmony of mind, body and spirit' (Campbell 1991, p. 8).

Nightingale introduced what I refer to as 'auditory modalities' as a form of nursing caring arts that foreshadowed the importance of sound and music as basic to health and nursing care:

> *The effect of music upon the sick has been scarcely at all noticed … wind instruments, including the human voice, and stringed instruments have … a beneficent effect. … while … such instruments as have no continuity of sound, have just the reverse. (p. 33)*

> *Noise … unnecessary noise, then, is the most cruel absence of care which can be inflicted either on the sick or well. (p. 27)*

> *Such unnecessary noise has undoubtedly induced or aggravated delirium in many cases. (p. 26)*

(1992 commemorative edition)

While Nightingale provided a blueprint for auditory modality, and while nursing has had access to auditory modalities across time, and even though nurses are often the ones who control and alter environmental noise, and who can influence system change and incorporate sound into routine practices of nursing, this basic nursing art and modality of care still remains largely an ad hoc practice, used by some individual nurses but not by others. It has yet to be systematically viewed as a caring art, and it is just beginning to be practiced and researched as basic to health, healing and self-care. Nevertheless, sound and music are increasingly emerging within a healing paradigm as a transpersonal caring–healing modality. We see evidence in the following ways.

Postmodern/transpersonal caring arts: auditory modality

Within contemporary thinking, we already see the intentional, conscious use of sound (for example, music, sounds of nature, wind, sea, chimes and chants, and familiar sounds) being made available for healing purposes and therapeutic ends. Music and sound act as catalysts to facilitate and enhance one's own inner healing and self-healing capacities; they evoke imagery, imagination and even transformation. Hospitals and healing practitioners such as massage therapists, physiotherapists, and nurses in hospitals, homes and clinics are consciously and intentionally using music to reduce stress and pain. Music and sound are used increasingly during chemotherapy to reduce nausea and vomiting, for elderly patients and those with Alzheimer's disease. Self-help tapes and compact discs frequently include meditative music, white noise, soothing sounds of whales, water and so forth, all designed to reframe one's inner consciousness, to release or relax. Some include overt or subliminal messages as affirmations, and verbal suggestions that tap into the unconscious mind and thought processes.

The latest approaches in this area are using what is referred to as 'deep sound' practices (Campbell 1984) for birthing, rebirthing, during life's major transitional events, and for persons who are unconscious or dying. The practices of sound to alter one's consciousness as a mystical and/or healing process have been used across time among indigenous people and religious monks and mystics, and in convents and sanctuaries, to enhance both spiritual and religious practices.

More recently, practices such as 'anointing one with sound' or 'giving a sonic bath' have arisen in work with persons going through the birth or death experience. The conscious use of sound is designed to select the appropriate tone and rhythm, to suit the desired state of consciousness, consistent with the experience and situation. For example, someone who was recovering from surgery would have music and sound designed to bring him or her into a more alert, engaged state of consciousness and to expand the senses. Someone who was going through a deathing experience would have music or sound which facilitated disengagement and the transition towards a more peaceful state. The field of music thanatology is increasingly being developed, using modalities such as the harp and voice to calm and enhance one's peaceful transition between life and death.

At a deep, human level, music transcends the science of sound and auditory modalities. Take, for example, the views of Lewis Thomas (1984), the research pathologist and former president and chancellor of the Memorial Sloan-Kettering Cancer Center in the USA. He frames the concept of music for the human senses much more poignantly than modern or postmodern medicine and nursing, and believes that:

> *The real meaning in music comes from tones only audible in the corner of the mind. (p. 13)*

> *If you are looking about for really profound mysteries, essential aspects of our existence for which neither the sciences nor the humanities can provide any sort of explanation, I suggest starting with music. The professional musicologists haven't the ghost of an idea about what music is, or why we make it and cannot be human without it, or even—and this is the telling point—how the human mind makes music on its own, before it is written down and played ... Nobody can explain it. It is a mystery, and thank goodness for that. (p. 162)* (Thomas 1984)

A number of readings and resources are suggested as ways in which to enrich one's thinking, understanding and practices relating to auditory modalities (see Further Reading, p. 234). While Nightingale's thinking prefaced sound therapy and music, it has emerged as part of a dominant modality for the new millennium, and remains essential to preserving the human experience and very existence.

Intentional conscious use of visual modalities

Premodern Nightingale caring arts 'from the margin'

Nightingale's words (1992 commemorative edition) on the importance of visual arts and beauty likewise foreshadowed what is emerging today as imagery and visual modalities. Here are her words on this topic, to help us reconsider the visual arts as caring arts emerging 'from the margin' of conventional practices into new, transpersonal modalities within the postmodern:

Variety and form of brilliancy of colour in objects ... are actual means of recovery. (p. 34)

The effect in sickness of beautiful objects, of variety of objects and especially of brilliancy of colour, is hardly at all appreciated. (p. 33)

A patient's bed should always be in the lightest spot in the room; and he should be able to see out of the window. (p. 47)

You will relieve, more effectually, unreasonable suffering ... by giving him something new to think of or to look at than by all the logic in the world. (p. 59)

I shall never forget the rapture of fever patients over a bunch of bright-coloured flowers ... (p. 34)

... affording them a pleasant view, a judicious variety as to flowers and pretty things ... a relief ... which a variety of objects before the eye affords ... (p. 35)

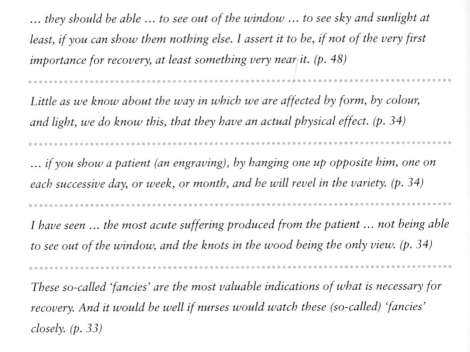

... they should be able ... to see out of the window ... to see sky and sunlight at least, if you can show them nothing else. I assert it to be, if not of the very first importance for recovery, at least something very near it. (p. 48)

Little as we know about the way in which we are affected by form, by colour, and light, we do know this, that they have an actual physical effect. (p. 34)

... if you show a patient (an engraving), by hanging one up opposite him, one on each successive day, or week, or month, and he will revel in the variety. (p. 34)

I have seen ... the most acute suffering produced from the patient ... not being able to see out of the window, and the knots in the wood being the only view. (p. 34)

These so-called 'fancies' are the most valuable indications of what is necessary for recovery. And it would be well if nurses would watch these (so-called) 'fancies' closely. (p. 33)

Postmodern/transpersonal caring arts: visual modality

Nightingale saw the importance of internal and external visual stimuli, light, color and beauty as effective agents of care and recovery that were integral to basic nursing. Today we increasingly see the conscious, intentional use of the visual modality, most overtly through the now popular use of imagery, healing arts and so forth. Visual images, both inner and outer, and transpersonal imagery serve now as rich, non-verbal approaches that can be introduced easily by nurses, family and friends, and can be self-regulated.

Both visual and imagery processes can be facilitated and guided by nurses and other health practitioners. When nurses engage in this form of caring arts, both individuals, the one-caring and the one-cared for, create a deeper and intersubjective relationship that can be transpersonal. This level of practice goes beyond conventional modern nursing care and can contribute to self-care healing practices.

Both external and internal visual objects and imaginary processes are increasingly used to affect emotions and alter physiology; a range of approaches related to visualization becomes a resource for gaining access to the imagination and the more subtle aspects of inner experience (Dossey et al 1995, p. 611). This caring art modality may involve all sensory modalities: visual, olfactory, tactile, gustatory, auditory and kinesthetic. Other examples of modalities that incorporate the notion of inner visualization include activities such as expressive journaling, dreamwork, storywork, personal narrative, and positive affirmations.

Nurses can integrate external and aesthetic visual approaches into their conventional care. Practitioners can more consciously and intentionally expand their practices to include visual, aesthetic healing space—light, color, form and texture—creating beauty in the immediate environment. This modality is also a natural venue for opening to and exploring the relational, transpersonal domain through the use of active imagery. General healing images and visualization include such processes as colors, sounds and the imaging of an inner guide. Likewise, the nurse or practitioner can serve as a guide. Nurses can effectively teach others to use visualization and imagery as a means of self-control, self-care, self-knowledge and self-healing. This modality may be used in any setting and at any time the person chooses; it is a non-invasive, non-intrusive, self-directed, self-regulatory approach that has no cost attached, yet has the potential to affect client outcomes (see Further Reading, p. 234).

In contemporary health settings, we see practices which consciously attend to, or introduce, beauty, works of art, aesthetics, light, color and nature in addition to formal imagery practices. These approaches, whether controlled and introduced internally or externally, help to calm, soothe, relax and potentiate images of harmony and wholeness of being. Nurses have used these modalities across time. Now they are being suggested as formal caring–healing modalities that the professional nurse and other healing practitioners will be expected to draw upon and incorporate into conventional and transpersonal practices.

Intentional conscious use of olfactory modalities

Premodern Nightingale caring arts from the margin'

At a time in our human history when fresh air and clean water can no longer be taken for granted, we find ourselves once again seeing the prophetic importance of Nightingale's insights into the importance of these basic nursing arts or caring modalities. In Nightingale's early vision she acknowledged the significance of the olfactory modality. We see from her words of 1859 how she addressed this modality:

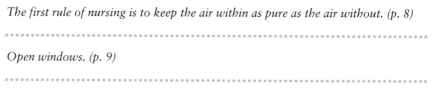

The first rule of nursing is to keep the air within as pure as the air without. (p. 8)

Open windows. (p. 9)

If the main function of a nurse is to maintain the air within the room as fresh as the air without ... then she should always be provided with ... an air test which indicates the organic matter of the air. (p. 10)

(1992 commemorative edition)

Postmodern/transpersonal caring arts: olfactory modality

Aromatherapy is perhaps the most commonly practiced version of this category, but the intentional conscious attention to breathwork, breathing, fresh air and inhalation–exhalation as meditative, relaxing and 'centering' approaches should also be considered. The development of the use of 'presence'—the cultivation of the transpersonal self, beyond the ego 'I'—through air, breathwork, breathing and selected aromas—all contribute to altering one's consciousness and moving toward more harmony, comfort, balance and wholeness.

The olfactory modality triggers other senses and carries what Marcel Proust (1925) suggested to be 'involuntary memories' of previous experiences (e.g. where the smell of entering one's garden takes one to an involuntary memory associated with another time). We can consciously and intentionally begin to pay attention to helping to create familiar scents in one's immediate setting by, for example, encouraging objects to be brought from one's home or surroundings. A child or adult might be provided with a comforting fragrance or familiar scent from, perhaps, a pillow case, or stuffed toy. The incorporation of symbolic, cleansing and purifying scents to patient care programs, individualized by the persons being cared for, now needs to be reconsidered as a basic intervention, instead of being ignored as unimportant or unhelpful.

At a broader community and environmental level we see that, from Nightingale onwards, this modality emphasizes the basic importance of clean air, water and environmental health in order for self, other, all living things, and the planet Earth to survive. While Nightingale's views were premodern with respect to these basics, we are now mandated to attend to them with renewed purpose and sophistication in this postmodern and post- postmodern time.

Lewis Thomas (1974) posed the olfactory receptor cell as one of the five wonders of the world. He noted that this cell was:

> ... located in the epithelial tissue high in the nose, sniffing the air for clues to the environment, the fragrance of friends, the smell of leaf smoke, breakfast, night-time, and bedtime, and a rose, even, it is said, the odor of sanctity. The cell that does all these things, firing off urgent messages into the deepest parts of the brain, switching on one strange unaccountable memory after another, is itself a proper 'brain cell', a certified neuron belonging to the brain but miles away out in the open air, nosing around the world. How it manages to make sense of what it senses, discriminating between jasmine and anything else non-jasmine with

infallibility, is one of the deep secrets of neurobiology. This would be wonder enough, but there is more. This population of brain cells, unlike any other neurons of the vertebrate central nervous system, turns itself over every few weeks; cells wear out, die, and are replaced by brand-new cells rewired to the same deep centers miles back in the brain, sensing and remembering the same wonderful smells.

Nurses and other practitioners can begin to reconsider the importance of this basic human sense modality in a variety of ways, as part of basic nursing arts. It is no wonder that we identify with Proust's involuntary memories of smell, in *Remembrance of Things Past* (1925), as he describes walking down the land and entering the gate to his home. It is not surprising that biofeedback therapists and others evoking relaxation ask their clients to conjure up the smell of blueberry muffins as they go into a relaxed state, in order to learn to control their biofeedback responses. They self-create the internal memory of smell as the starting point for memory, for remembering, for returning home, so to speak, to a quiet, safe space within.

Nurses and others are increasingly using essential oils and aromatherapy as part of their practices. Since aromatherapy is the most common example of a formal modality in this category, a number of books on the subject are included in the Further Reading list (p. 234).

Intentional conscious use of tactile modality

Premodern Nightingale caring arts 'from the margin'

While the tactile modality is fundamental to nursing and nursing care, only recently has serious attention been given to touch and the different ways of considering the importance of touch as a caring art. In my research on Nightingale, I could not find any direct references to the use of touch, but she does indicate the use of the tactile as part of basic nursing arts. This tactile reference was with regard to bathing:

*Take a rough towel, dip one corner in … hot water—if a little spirit be added to it,
it will be more effectual—and then rub as if you were rubbing the towel into your
skin with your fingers. (p. 53)*

*And you can really keep yourself cleaner with a tumbler of water and a rough
towel and rubbing, than … without rubbing. (p. 54)*

(1992 commemorative edition)

Postmodern/transpersonal caring arts: tactile modality

While touch is an ancient form of healing and has been practiced intentionally across cultures, Nightingale did not explicitly address touch per se.
Nevertheless, today we see formal touch modalities, ranging from non-
contact touch to intentional touch, therapeutic massage and manipulation.
Some of these different modes of intentional conscious use of touch have
been identified and defined by Keegan (1995, p. 540). The different modes
and definitions of touch are included in Box 14.1.

Excluding therapeutic touch, all body touch therapies involve actual
physical contact. Touch is one of the most easily used caring arts modalities; it can help to integrate and harmonize, and to provide comfort,
wholeness and integrity and even a sense of safety. But touch can also be
used in a way that is not comforting, and can be less than therapeutic.

Touch is a basic human sense mode and basic human need. There are
indications that some elderly people, for example, are 'starved for human
touch' and experience what is referred to as 'skin hunger'. The same is true
from self-reports of persons with AIDS; they talk about the lack of human
touch and how healing it can be for someone to just touch them, hold their
hand or hug them.

The sensory use of touch as a stimulus for persons who are sensory
deprived is not to be overlooked as a basic caring art. The touching of
fabrics and textiles, and the feeling of different object shapes, of sculptures

Box 14.1 Touch modes and definitions (From 'Holistic Nursing' by B M Dossey, L Keegan, C E Guzzetta, L G Kolkmeier © 1995. Reprinted with permission from Aspen Publishers, Inc., Gaithersburg.)

Acupressure: the application of finger and/or thumb pressure to specific sites along the body's energy meridians for the purpose of relieving tension and reestablishing the flow of energy along the meridian lines.

Body therapy and/or touch therapy: the broad range of techniques that a practitioner uses with the hands on or near the body to assist the recipient toward optimal function.

Caring touch: touch done with a genuine interest in the other person [along with authentic engagement and concern]. (Author's parenthesis: modification of definition.)

Centering: a process of going within to create an 'inner sense of self-relatedness that can be thought of as a place of inner being, a place of quietude within oneself where one can feel truly integrated, unified, and focused.'

Energy meridian: an energy circuit or line of force. Eastern theories describe meridian lines flowing vertically through the body with culminating points on the feet, hands and head. (These points are depicted in Alex Grey's *Sacred Mirrors* art series, entitled Psychic Energy System (see Plate 9A).)

Foot reflexology: the application of pressure to points on the feet that correspond to other parts of the body.

Intention: the motivation or reason for touching; (one's intention in this framework is consciously, intentionally directed toward, for example, wholeness, healing, and comfort).

Procedural touch: touch done to diagnose, monitor or treat the illness itself; touch that focuses on the end result of curing the illness or preventing further complications.

Shiatsu: the use of the thumb and/or heel of the hand for deep-pressure work along the energy meridian lines.

Therapeutic massage: the use of the hands to apply pressure and motion on the skin and underlying muscle of the recipient for the purposes of physical and psychological relaxation, improvement of circulation, relief of sore muscles, and other therapeutic effects.

Therapeutic touch: a specific technique of centering intention used while the practitioner moves the hands through a recipient's energy field for the purpose of assessment and treatment of energy field imbalance.

and natural items such as leaves, pine cones and flowers, can be important touch stimuli for someone who is sensory deprived.

The intentional conscious use of touch, massage and therapeutic touch are now being used as part of holistic and transpersonal practices. During the early part of the modern nursing era, touch and massage were used more systematically as a nursing caring art. 'Back rubs' were a common aspect of basic care and a bedtime preparation for entire patient groups up until about the late 1960s. With the advent of new technology, medical interventions and increased adherence to institutional procedures, the basic caring arts including touch and massage were no longer considered to be essential to standard nursing care. Caring touch was substituted by increasing nurse practitioner skills, such as the use of the stethoscope, the undertaking of total physical assessments, engaging in intravenous administrations and respiratory care, and monitoring telemetry. These intersected with the move toward nursing science and the science behind procedures and skills. This shift left the basic caring arts behind, including touch modalities. They now need to be reintegrated, and are re-emerging as mature caring–healing practices. The public is also more demanding of touch therapies, both in and out of institutions, for self-care, relaxation, health-promoting approaches and therapeutic treatment modalities.

Some of the caring touch approaches, such as therapeutic touch, acu-pressure, shiatsu and healing touch, are energy-based therapeutics. These particular approaches involve the conscious intent to help or heal; they are used to decrease anxiety, relieve pain and facilitate the healing process. Therapeutic touch was developed by Krieger at New York University, utilizing Rogers' nursing theory of the human energy field (Krieger 1979, Rogers 1970). Since then, Quinn (1996) and others have been involved in additional study, teaching, practice and research of this modality.

Healing touch, like therapeutic touch, is based upon the concept of an energy field, and is intentionally directed towards physical, emotional, mental and spiritual health and healing (Mentgen, Trapp & Bulbrook

1994). The American Holistic Nurses' Association offers a certificate program in this modality.

While therapeutic massage, reflexology and other forms of touch are increasingly used in nursing and other fields, this section is not intended to develop and describe the various modalities. (See Further Reading, p. 234, for more information on these.) Rather, the purpose here is to emphasize that touch, both general and specific, is a contemporary caring arts modality, consistent with transpersonal caring and healing.

Each practitioner is challenged to be cognizant and skilled in the various modalities of choice, talent and interest, recognizing that mature caring–healing practices incorporate a range of these sensory-based modalities that are yet to be fully integrated into nursing education and practice. The emerging transpersonal perspective attends to the range of touch modalities and/or assists in coordinating these options into existing plans of care.

Intentional conscious use of gustatory modalities

Premodern Nightingale caring arts 'from the margin'

Nightingale addresses this basic sense modality as being integral to nursing care. The attention to food, drink and taste, and to the symbolic meaning of this sense, was part of her instructions for care:

> ... there is nothing yet discovered which is a substitute to the English patient for his cup of tea; he can take it when he can take nothing else, and he often can't take anything else if he has it not. (p. 43)

> You cannot diet a patient from a book, you cannot make up the human body as you would make up a prescription. (p. 41)

> ... being so badly cooked that he always left them untouched. (p. 40)

The patient's stomach must be its own chemist. (p. 42)

... the conviction that the craving for variety in the starving eye, is just as desperate as that for food in the starving stomach, and tempts the famishing creature in either case to steal for its satisfaction.

(1992 commemorative edition)

Nightingale addressed the basics of feeding patients and some general rules regarding food, ways of serving it and conditions for increasing the likelihood of eating. Today, there is much necessary attention paid to the gustatory sense and its relationship to diet, nutrition and a basic healthy lifestyle, whether sick or well.

Postmodern/transpersonal caring arts: gustatory modality

The current focus on diet, food, texture, aroma, appearance, atmosphere and environment all come into play within the postmodern considerations. The sensual experiences associated with food preparation, and the notion of treating and eating food as a sacred event, are parts of the transpersonal awareness related to this modality. Honoring food, taking what one needs and eating what one takes without waste, is part of being consciously and intentionally aware of the politics of food—knowing that it is not through lack of abundance that part of the world goes hungry but through unfair distribution and waste.

Within the transpersonal, food, eating and the gustatory sense mode become part of our conscious awareness of nurturing ourselves at all levels. Healing nutrition and dietary selections and changes are becoming active self-care approaches for a variety of health and illness conditions, from cancer care to staying fit.

Within the transpersonal, we open ourselves to the deeper meaning of food, to our connection with Mother Earth and the cycles of light and dark, and to earth, air, fire and water as the elemental forces providing us with nutrients and conveniences for foods and their preparation.

Recognizing one's relationship with food, and food's many diverse meanings and associations, becomes a fundamental caring art. Personalizing tastes and habits for individual care can make a difference to one's intake, to the nourishment associated with the food, and to the eating experience. The care of our bodies through food and taste, with all food's associations and meanings, increases both our physical and spiritual capacities.

Under Further Reading (p. 235), a number of books are suggested to augment understanding and appreciation of this modality as a basic element of the caring arts.

Intentional use of mental–cognitive modalities

Premodern Nightingale caring arts 'from the margin'

While today there are a variety of theories and approaches within this category, Nightingale foreshadowed the importance of this caring art as part of basic nursing. The following statements about this area are taken from her writings:

Help the sick to vary their thoughts ... Sick children may prefer a story to be told to them. (p. 32)

You will relieve, more effectually, unreasonable suffering ... by giving him something new to think of ... than by all the logic in the world. (p. 59)

Always ... give complete attention and full consideration. (p. 28)

... in very many cases, the imagination in disease is far more active and vivid than it is in health. (p. 28)

You have no idea what the craving of the sick, with undiminished power of thinking ... is to hear of good. (p. 58)

(1992 commemorative edition)

Postmodern/transpersonal caring arts: mental–cognitive modalities

Nightingale's consideration of the importance of the mind and the imagination through story, attention and good news set the scene for what have become today's transpersonal practices and extended caring arts. These extended practices can be translated as formal visualization, imagery, cognitive therapy, dreamwork, the use of humor, play, story, literature, poetry and art, positive affirmations, expressive journaling, dialogue and teaching, including thought and 'no-thought' approaches aimed at gaining silence and solitude, and contemplative and meditative practices.

This range of modalities overlaps with consciousness modalities, and will not be explored here other than to mention the unlimited aspects of this area of caring arts and nursing modalities. It is important to highlight that the area has been relatively untapped by nurses until recent times. Yet nurses have continuous relationships with patients and families across the life span, in and out of institutions. They have freedom to develop and incorporate these caring–healing modalities in ways yet to be imagined but waiting to be discovered. Some suggested readings are given in Further Reading (p. 235) to assist nurses in this area.

Intentional conscious use of kinesthetic modalities

Premodern Nightingale caring arts 'from the margin'

Nightingale had some interesting views, views that were ahead of her time, on the importance of basic body–mind interactions and the ability of the body to have its own effect. Her words in 1859 could be spoken today:

> Volumes are now written and spoken about the effect of the mind upon the body. Much of it is true. But I wish a little more was thought of the effect of the body on the mind. (p. 34)

People say the effect is only on the mind. It is no such thing. The effect is on the body, too. (p. 34)

. . . .

Poisoning by the skin is no less certain than poisoning by the mouth—only it is slower in its operation. (p. 53)

. . . .

The amount of relief and comfort experienced by the sick after the skin has been carefully washed and dried, is one of the commonest observations made at a sick bed. (p. 53)

(1992 commemorative edition)

Postmodern/transpersonal caring arts, kinesthetic modalities

It is interesting that this line of thinking coincides with some recent developments discussed in the chapter on the postmodern–transpersonal body (Ch. 10). Within a contemporary postmodern paradigm, focus on kinesthetics of the body-physical ranges from basic skin care, which Nightingale addressed, to deep massage and deep cellular tissue work such as Rolfing, to movement, dance, yoga and Tai Chi. This modality also overlaps with touch therapies. The bodywork fields, such as applied kinesiology, chiropractic, Feldenkrais work, Jin shin Jyutsu, polarity work, Reiki and Trager work, are just some of the more developed and practiced body therapies within the kinesthetic category.

The use of smooth, flowing body movement, dance and rhythmic flow are increasingly being incorporated into therapeutic and formal treatment programs. (See Table 14.1 for a list of these current approaches and their primary purpose and function.) Nurses and other practitioners can incorporate some of the techniques into their caring arts work, or develop skills and additional training as a formal practitioner of one or more of these modalities.

Table 14.1 Additional touch therapies (From 'Holistic Nursing' by B M Dossey, L Keegan, C E Guzzetta, L G Kolkmeier © 1995. Reprinted with permission from Aspen Publishers, Inc., Gaithersburg.)

Therapy	Originator	Primary purpose and function
Applied kinesiology	George Goodheart	Focuses on the relationship of muscle strength and energy flow. The theory is that if muscles are strong, then circulation and other vital functions are also strong.
Chiropractic	D D Palmer	Based on the alignment of spinal vertebrae. This therapy involves manipulations to restore natural alignment.
Feldenkrais	Moshe Feldenkrais	Purpose is to give the client gentle manipulations to heighten awareness of the body. As awareness increases, clients can make more informed choices about how to move the body in daily situations.
Jin shin jyutsu	Master Jiro Murai of Japan in early 1900s	A milder form of acupressure that involves pressure along the eight extra acupuncture meridians.
Kofutu touch healing	Frank Homan	System developed in the early 1970s when a series of symbols for use in touch came to the originator during meditation. It is called 'Kofutu' for the symbols and 'touch' healing because the auras of the healer and recipient must touch. This therapy uses higher-consciousness energy symbols for the purpose of self-development and spiritual healing.
Lomi	R K Hall, R K Heckler	Directs attention to current muscle tension to aid learning of postural alignment to enhance free flow of the body's physical and emotional energies.
Polarity	Randolph Stone	Repatterns energy flow in the individual by rebalancing positive and negative charges. The practitioner places finger or whole hand on parts of the client's body of opposite charge for the purpose of facilitating energy balancing where it is needed. Through these contacts, with the help of pressure and rocking movements, energy can reorganize and reorder itself.
MariEL	Ethel Lombardi	A 1980s variation of Reiki.
Neuromuscular release		Practitioner moves the limbs into and away from the body to assist the client in learning to 'let go' for the purpose of enhanced circulation and emotional release.

Table 14.1 *(cont'd)*		
Therapy	**Originator**	**Primary purpose and function**
Reiki	2500-year-old Buddhist practice lost and rediscovered in late 1800s	Reiki means 'universal life energy'. A touch technique in which the practitioner places hands in one of 12 positions on the recipient's body to direct healing energy to those sites.
Rolfing	Ida P Rolf	Purpose is to help the client establish deep structural relationships within the body that manifest themselves via a symmetry and balanced function when the body is in an upright position. Technique involves deep muscle manipulation.
Trager	Milton Trager	Limbs and often the whole body are rocked rhythmically to aid relaxation of the muscles to promote an optimal flow of blood, lymph, nerve impulses and energy.

Intentional conscious use of 'caring consciousness' as modality

Premodern Nightingale caring arts 'from the margin'

In this last modality within the caring arts framework which can be traced back to Nightingale for its origins and blueprint for the future, I turn to consciousness itself. Within the transpersonal framework, one's consciousness affects one's being, one's relationship with self and other, and one's intentionality. Consciousness, as developed earlier in this book, is posited to carry energy which can be transmitted and communicated between people. One's consciousness is capable of changing a transpersonal field, within a given 'caring moment'. We find traces of this insight in Nightingale's discussion of the nurse's presence and awareness, and how this affects the patient:

> It is fair to say that this death was attributed to fright. It was the result of a long whispered conversation within sight of the patient. (p. 26)

Such unnecessary noise has undoubtedly induced or aggravated delirium in many cases. (p. 26)

These things are not fancy. If we consider that, with sick as with well, every thought decomposes some nervous matter—that decomposition as well as recomposition of nervous matter is always going on. (p. 28)

If a patient has to see not only to his own but also to his nurse's ... perseverance or readiness, or calmness, to any or all of these things, he is far better without that nurse than with her. (p. 31)

(1992 commemorative edition)

Already we see glimpses indicating that the nurse's presence and consciousness, attitude and behavior can affect the patient, for better or for worse.

Postmodern/transpersonal caring arts: caring consciousness—being, presence

As discussed within Chapter 9 on transpersonal self and the transpersonal caring moment, the role of consciousness, intentionality and presence was developed theoretically. The theory can be translated into an actual caring art that affects the healing and well-being of both self and other. One can identify and integrate many modes that can affect one's caring–healing consciousness through self-applied practices and activities. These self-practices, in turn, can be authentically integrated into one's professional practice.

The concept of presence has been explored in the nursing literature. McKivergin & Daubenmire (1994, pp. 65–81) identified three levels of presence:

1. *Physical presence:* 'being there' for the other. This implies actual body-to-body contact. It may involve seeing, examining, touching,

doing, hearing, hugging and similar physically present contact (Keegan 1995). Much of routine nursing occurs at this level.

2. *Psychological presence:* 'being with' the other. This involves mind-to-mind connection. The therapeutic use of self, and using self to create a caring–healing milieu, takes nursing beyond the routine level toward a more authentic caring presence. The skills include having conscious intention to be available to another; together with a basic helping relationship and communication skills, such as active listening, congruence, unconditional regard and non-judgmental acceptance.

3. *Therapeutic presence.* This level of presence is most closely aligned with caring consciousness, mindfulness, intentionality and transpersonal caring; it incorporates centering, meditating, intentionality, at-one-ment, intuitive connecting, openness, communion, loving and connecting. This level of presence can be translated into transpersonal presence.

Overall, in this caring art, *one's being is the modality*. It invites the culmination of all the other modes and manifests itself in a given moment, in any relationship, in any caring art, or mode of practice. The cultivation of a 'caring consciousness' as a way of 'being', and as a way of being authentically 'present', requires focused practice and development.

Transpersonal presence and a caring consciousness can be cultivated through any and all of the modalities addressed above. It can be cultivated through meditation, deep relaxation exercises, hypnosis, positive affirmations, imagery, visualization, solitude, cultivation of mindfulness, and being in the moment; through the practice of self-love, compassion, peace through yoga, centering prayer, other forms of prayer and contemplative practice; and through the use of poetry, humanities, literature, story, ritual, movement, touch and bodywork.

The cultivation of transpersonal self (to become aware of one's consciousness and intentionality) requires one to develop lifelong, sustainable practices. As one does this, one enters the spiritual path toward transformation and healing. In turn, one becomes part of a collective group of practitioners who are increasingly helping to shift from the modern mindset towards one that is actively directed toward caring, peace, love, and healing as a way of being present to self, other and life itself.

Discussion of postmodern/ transpersonal caring arts

Within the context of the model of transpersonal caring–healing and discussions related to ontological competencies and caring–healing modalities, we can consider Nightingale's advice as if for the first time. We can listen to its timelessness and timeliness, and recognize its significance for a maturing nursing transpersonal paradigm—now seen and heard from an emerging cosmology, with the benefits of a century of evolving consciousness.

Reframing some of the nursing arts or acts which have been taken for granted presents a broader, more complex and more complete explanation of phenomena and practices; the postmodern slant brings new meaning to the modern. It helps us see how underdeveloped nursing has been in actualizing its own caring–healing practices, since many of the modalities have been excluded from nursing or, in some instances, excluded from the human consciousness of the modern era during the 20th century.

It is crucial for nursing and health professionals to recognize that the transpersonal caring–healing modalities are used commonly by the public. Nurses and other practitioners are engaged in these practices at varying levels of sophistication and development. Some are treated as techniques to be added to the existing Era I and II/Paradigm I and II practices. Some alternative practitioners are engaged in these practices as healing arts committed to transformation and healing, rather than to treatment and cure.

One of the dangers at this juncture is that nurses and others will incorporate these approaches as technical (medical) interventions, without grounding in an ethical, philosophical, theoretical and scientific framework. They could then become co-opted by mainstream medicine, or be excluded altogether, or considered tangential to traditional 'legitimate' modalities that are medically derived, as opposed to being informed by 'legitimate' caring–healing wholeness models residing with the sacred feminine archetype paradigm of nursing's historical roots.

Within the Era III/Paradigm III framework of this book, what was once considered routine physical care in the modern framework now becomes transformed care of embodied spirit, translating otherwise ordinary care into sacred acts—life-generating processes whereby conscious, intentional caring–healing modalities for the whole person fall within the domain of nursing while, paradoxically, transcending nursing.

Within the philosophy of transpersonal caring, consciousness and energy take on new meanings. Sarter points out that, in reconsidering nursing therapeutics (or caring–healing modalities) within a consciousness paradigm, care can be described and classified according to the level of consciousness that it influences. She hypothesizes that those interventions or modalities that operate at the 'higher frequency, higher consciousness levels will be of the greater influence, since they will affect all the lower levels of consciousness that are operative for the client' (Sarter 1987 pp. 6–7). She uses the examples of touch or massage, which may be found to operate primarily at the physical and what she calls the pranic levels of consciousness. (Pranic is a Sanskrit term meaning 'breath 'or 'life'; in Ayurvedic medicine it is 'organic energy', vital organizing energy that regulates life processes and permeates and integrates the living organism; 'pranic' consciousness knows what it needs to maintain life processes.)

Sarter proposes that visualization or imagery would intervene primarily at the level of mental consciousness; meditation or prayer would intervene at the spiritual level of consciousness, thereby permeating all levels below it. She proposes that a vast number of traditional and more recently developed therapeutic measures could be explained within this framework, according to the organization of consciousness energy and its interactions and effects.

Sarter's ideas are intriguing and are possibly consistent with the framework I am proposing, with further clarification and exploration. However, I am proposing that the higher-frequency energy of the caring/loving consciousness and the intentionality of the practitioner also affect the lower-frequency energy system within a given interaction of coming together into a shared energy field, or field of consciousness. The energy consciousness of the practitioner would have the potential to change the whole field of energy consciousness in a given caring moment.

In this transpersonal framework, different caring–healing modalities may be operating at different levels of consciousness in the client. If a person is viewed as an embodied spirit, possessing a soul, then it is possible that any one of the caring modalities may be effectively permeating other levels of consciousness.

With this line of thinking, could it be that the nurse's touch triggers involuntary memories, archetypal, deep connections that reside in the cells, the muscles and the psyche? Could it be that touch can occur at levels deeper than the physical level, that touch triggers a whole symbolic chain of memories from childhood and beyond? Could it be that such a paradigm calls forth the concept of sacred touch, sacred presence and sacred movement and being, that we are touching souls, not just bodies?

Nightingale's description of working with the living body, as the temple of God's spirit, takes on a whole new meaning within the transpersonal context. Nightingale made it explicit that nursing deals with the human spirit and that nursing acts are the art from which patients are enabled to spiritually develop. It is the spirit of our consciousness which informs our practices. If the practitioner holds a caring consciousness and intentionality toward sacred healing, harmony and wholeness in each art or act, then a healing context is created as a sacred space for each caring occasion. Each act thereby potentiates healing.

These examples in no way preclude practices that are already common, such as emotional, expressive and relational work, as developed in my earlier work as 'carative factors'. In this framework, I am trying to help us to see again what is already inscribed in our work but which lies dormant and underdeveloped on the margins of both modern medicine and nursing practice.

These so-called postmodern/transpersonal professional caring–healing modalities may even be considered in some instances to be premodern. However, they are now located within a different and emerging paradigm and within a new cosmology. They flow from a spiritual path of humans developing and evolving in their consciousness and intentionality, and from those ontological competencies of being. They build upon the cultivation of presence, caring and healing consciousness, and on intentionality of healing and wholeness. These ontological dimensions of 'being at-one-ment' in a caring moment, fully embodied yet with transcendent possibilities, become the foundation for transpersonal practice now and in the future.

Postmodern/transpersonal awareness can transform technology and the dominant paradigm of medicine as well as that of nursing. When considering advanced caring–healing arts within a transpersonal paradigm, and from within a sacred archetype cosmology, one can begin to see that the ontological competencies and advanced caring–healing modalities are consistent with some of the foundational approaches of Nightingale's model and metaparadigm for nursing, yet to be actualized. As Nightingale put it, nursing arts are maybe among the most comprehensive and difficult of all arts. The artistry by which nursing draws upon nature and the life spirit often captures, expresses and reflects humanity and life in all its various and diverse forms.

During nursing's modern rise, these aspects of nursing became subsumed under medical care and institutional demands. The irony is that these are the very modalities that are now needed to transform health care for the next century. These so-called early premodern nursing therapeutics were lost to nursing's advancing models for scientific practice. As nursing arts of caring and healing are reintegrated into professional nursing education and practice, nursing indeed becomes an *ontological artistry,* symbolizing and actualizing the sacred archetypal acts for wholeness and healing.

Ontological caring–healing competencies—the artistry of the modalities suggested above—all provide access to *consciousness.* They tap into feelings, emotions, inner processes, imagery, intuition, and into the deep center—the higher/deeper self—with increasing access to higher, universal consciousness. The advanced practitioner in this model becomes an expert in the ontology of caring and healing arts.

Such a model provides very different consequences for academe and clinical settings. Shepherd (1993) referred to this kind of reconstructing as 'lifting the veil', ushering in the sacred feminine ontology as a way of being in transpersonal relationships. Such attention to ontology, consciousness, energy, caring ethic and caring arts as proposed in this book is consistent with Shepherd's (1993) concepts and directions and is a new guide to all of us in our work. These directions, identified by Shepherd, return us to a sacred feminine archetype that includes:

- *Feelings:* for example, advocating research and inquiry motivated by love and caring; bringing feelings back into our discourse in classrooms and in clinical settings.

- *Receptivity:* listening to self, other and nature, and receiving, remembering and relearning about ourselves and our being-in-the-world.
- *Subjectivity/intersubjectivity:* discovering ourselves through experiences, dialogue and experiments with different laws of living.
- *Mulitiplicity:* considering our webs of interaction, healing webs and caring communities, and increasing diversity in being and knowing, living and evolving as spiritual beings.
- *Nurturing:* reclaiming nursing as the sacred archetype for nourishing and bringing warmth and beauty into our personal, inner lives and our surroundings; welcoming the feminine; providing comfort, ease, solitude and safe, healing space; nurturing ideas in addition to nurturing an expanding consciousness.
- *Cooperating:* relating and bringing harmony and wholeness into our acts, relationships and environments.
- *Intuiting:* developing artistry of being; using the imagination, and constructing a future of what might be, rather than conforming to what is.
- *Relatedness:* forming a vision of wholeness, connectedness; relational ontology of being, knowing and doing.
- *Loving and caring:* developing the foundation of being for professional practice; the source of inspiration, compassion, commitment and energy.
- *Peace:* within this postmodern clearing for new possibilities of transpersonal caring, we not only reach for caring and healing but also offer a hope for peace. Within a different cosmology and consciousness, we reach an ethical responsibility to seek peace and to remember the sacred feminine for healing.

This perspective provides a framework and pathway whereby we might journey toward the 'medicine man' and 'medicine woman' healer in us all (Shepherd 1993).

Whether nursing chooses to advance within its own mature paradigm and transform its caring–healing practices from the modern emphasis on body-physical care to the postmodern/transpersonal embodied spirit care-as-sacred act, or whether it remains within the biomedical Era I and Era II paradigms for its advancement, is a decision that is yet to be made by mainstream nursing. Nursing is a profession and discipline at a crossroads in its maturation and in its paradigm choices. If nursing does not make the choice for transformation and maturation within its own paradigm, then I predict that another professional group will emerge to meet the needs of the public. If this happened, nursing would remain on the margin of a transformed system, either partially practicing nursing, or else relegating to the technical Era I and II/Paradigm I and II practices.

At the disciplinary level, nursing science is heading towards Paradigm III models for its inquiry and scholarship, consistent with all branches of knowledge in the academy of learning. The hope is that academic nursing will transform its educational-practice models to prepare practitioners to practice the more complete paradigm of nursing, one that not only is able to integrate medical and technological aspects into its practices, but also transforms them along with a totally new view of advanced nursing practice. This position does not preclude other nurses practicing at different points on the evolutionary continuum, moving towards transpersonal caring and healing.

FURTHER READING

Auditory modalities

Campbell D 1984 Introduction to the musical brain. MMB Music, St Louis
Campbell D (ed) 1991 Music: physician for times to come. Quest, Wheaton
Campbell D (ed) 1992 Music and miracles. Quest, Wheaton
Halpern S, Savary L 1985 Sound health: music and sounds that make us whole. Harper & Row, San Francisco
Homel P M 1979 Through music to the self. Shambhala, Boston
McClellan R 1979 Music and altered states of consciousness. Dromenon 2:3–5
Thomas L 1984 Late night thoughts on listening to Mahler's ninth symphony. Bantam, New York

Visual modalities and imagery

Achterberg J 1985 Imagery in healing. Shambhala, Boston
Achterberg J, Dossey B, Kolkmeier L G 1994 Rituals of healing. Bantam, New York
Dossey B 1995 Imagery. In: Dossey B M, Keegan L, Guzzetta C, Kolkmeier L G Holistic nursing, 2nd edn, Aspen, Gaithersburg, pp 609–666
Gablik S 1991 The re-enchantment of art. Thames & Hudson, New York
Gadamer H G 1986 The relevance of the beautiful and other essays. Translated by Walker N, Bernasconi R (eds) Cambridge University Press, New York
McNiff S 1992 Art as medicine. Shambhala, Boston
Nightingale F 1859 (1992 commemorative edn) Notes on nursing. J P Lippincott, Philadelphia

Olfactory modality and aromatherapy

Nightingale F 1859 (1992 commemorative edn) Notes on nursing. J P Lippincott, Philadelphia
Proust M 1925 Remembrance of things past. Random House, New York
Thomas L 1974 The lives of a cell. Bantam, New York
Walji H 1996 The healing power of aromatherapy. Prima Publications, Rocklin

Tactile modality and a caring touch

Barnett K 1972 A survey of the current utilization of touch by health team personnel with hospitalized patients. International Journal of Nursing Studies 9:195–209
Bottorff J 1991 A methodological review and evaluation of research on nurse–patient touch. In: Anthology on caring, Chinn P L (ed) National League for Nursing, New York, pp. 303–343
Hover D 1995 Healing touch. Delmar, New York
Keegan L 1995 Touch. In: Dossey B M, Keegan L, Guzzetta C E, Kolkmeier L G (authors) Holistic nursing: a handbook for practice. Aspen, Gaithersburg, pp. 539–567
Krieger D 1979 The therapeutic touch. Prentice-Hall, Englewood Cliffs
Krieger D 1981 Foundations for holistic health nursing practices: the renaissance nurse. J B Lippincott, Philadelphia
Kunz K, Kunz B 1980 The complete guide to foot reflexology. Prentice-Hall, Englewood Cliffs

Mentgen J, Trapp-Bulbrook M J 1994 Healing touch. North Carolina Center for
    Healing Touch, Carraboro
McCorkle R 1974 Effects of touch on seriously ill patients. Nursing Research
    pp 125–132
Quinn J 1992 The nurse as healing environment. Holistic Nursing Practice 6(4):26–35
Rozema H 1986 Touch needs of the elderly. Nursing Homes, pp. 42–43
Simon S 1974 Please touch! How to combat skin hunger in our schools. Scholastic
    Teacher, pp. 22–25
Rogers M 1970 A theoretical basis of nursing. F A Davis, Philadelphia

Gustatory modality

David M 1991 Nourishing wisdom: a new understanding of eating. Bell Tower,
    New York
Keegan L 1995 Nutrition, exercise, and movement. In: Dossey B, Keegan L,
    Guzzetta C, Kolkmeier L G (authors) Holistic nursing: a handbook for practice.
    Aspen, Gaithersburg
Keegan L 1996 Healing nutrition. Delmar, Albany, p. 540

Mental cognitive modalities

Burns D 1990 Feeling good: the new mood therapy. New American Library,
    New York
Kolkmeier L G 1995 Cognitive therapy. In: Dossey B, Keegan L, Guzzetta C,
    Kolkmeier L G 1995 Holistic nursing: a handbook for practice. Aspen,
    Gaithersburg
Schuyler D 1991 A practical guide to cognitive therapy. W W North, New York

Caring consciousness—being, presence

Achterberg J, Dossey B, Kolkmeier L G 1994 Rituals of healing. Bantam, New York
Burch S 1994 Consciousness: an analysis of the concept. Journal of Holistic Nursing
    12(1):101–116
Gaut D (ed) 1992 The presence of caring in nursing. National League for Nursing,
    New York
Gilje F 1992. Being there: an analysis of the concept of presence. In: Gaut D (ed) 1992
    The presence of caring in nursing. National League for Nursing, New York,
    pp. 53–67
Keegan L 1995 Touch. In: Dossey B, Keegan L, Guzzetta C, Kolkmeier L 1995
    Holistic nursing: a handbook for practice. Aspen, Gaithersburg
McKevergin M, Daubenmire J 1994 The essence of therapeutic presence. Journal of
    Holistic Nursing 12(1):65–81
Montgomery C 1992 The spiritual connection: nurses' perceptions of the experience
    of caring. In: Gaut D (ed) The presence of caring in nursing. National League for
    Nursing, New York
Newman M 1994 Health as expanding consciousness. National League for Nursing,
    New York
Watson J 1988b Nursing: human science and human care. National League for
    Nursing, New York

15

An interlude: the Zen of bedmaking

To see a World in a Grain of Sand, and a Heaven in a Wild Flower, Hold Infinity in the palm of your hand, and Eternity in an hour.

(Blake 1796, in: Norton 1975, p. 555)

Look at the ordinary bed in which a patient lies. If I were looking out for an example in order to show what not to do, I should take the specimen of an ordinary bed ...

(Nightingale 1859, in: 1992 commemorative edition)

As we pause to consider the importance of each caring act within a transpersonal framework of conscious intentionality, and as we honor each caring act and each caring moment, let us consider the following as a somewhat playful but neverthless powerful reminder of how each moment and each act contains the whole universe of caring and healing. In the words of Nightingale, 'take the specimen of an ordinary bed' (1992 commemorative edition).

Nursing from premodern times onward has been associated with bed and bedmaking, and all the positive and negative connotations associated with those words. For example, one may look at a bed and see it as an object, and bedmaking as a technical procedure, usually one relegated to an assistant. Yet it remains a standard part of all nursing curricula, a must for all students to learn.

Perhaps another way for nursing to consider the bed, whether the nurse deals with bedmaking or not, is to view bed and bedmaking as a metaphor for any nursing art or any caring act. Consider the 'Zen of bedmaking'. By this I mean that 'bed' stands as a vehicle for an expanded consciousness of all; the bed and all its meanings contain the absolute universe.

The word 'Zen' has its ancient roots in Sanskrit and means 'contemplation, meditation' (Campbell 1972, p. 131). Rather than seeing bed as tangential or trivial, one may look at bed and see it as a sacred space. The bed, or any caring act or nursing art, stands alone in this example as a single statement, symbolizing beauty, simplicity, elegance, wholeness; it is an invitation to comfort, safety, privacy, rest, recovery and a place for healing to occur.

There is a story, told by a Zen master, about the teachings of Buddha. The story is told this way (Campbell 1972, p. 133):

During one of Buddha's teachings, his message was contained in a single gesture: holding up a single lotus. That simple gesture contained the whole message. However, only one member of his audience caught the message. Buddha, noticing his comprehension, gave him a knowing nod, and then continued with a verbal teaching for his audience, since they still required a teaching to 'get' the meaning.

With this story, Campbell reminded us that we are so entrapped in a net of ideas that we fail to grasp the importance of a single act, a single event— yet each act contains the entire universe, if we 'get' it. In this instance, bed as metaphor stands for a nursing act but also points beyond it, capturing a universe of caring (or non-caring). Yet, if I were to hold up the word 'bed', would we 'get it'? Are we so entrapped by our stereotypes, by our role definitions and professionalization, that we miss a single caring moment that carries the whole?

What if I were to hold up the word 'bed' and ask for its meaning in a Zen sense, as Nightingale put it, as a single specimen of a nursing event? And what if you really 'got it', like the student of Buddha—if indeed, the object or event is experienced simply in, and for, and as, itself? Then 'such a moment of sheer aesthetic arrest throws the viewer back for an instant upon his own existence ... for he too, simply *is* ... a vehicle of consciousness (Campbell 1972, p. 141).

Within the caring consciousness proposed here, the Zen of nursing requires us to reconsider nursing skills for new reasons, and to reframe nursing art/acts within an entirely different framework of meaning and significance—'seeing the whole in each part.' Indeed, can we open ourselves up again to the freshness and miracle of seeking and 'see a World in a Grain of Sand, and a Heaven in a Wild Flower?' (Blake 1796, in: Norton 1975).

If so, then there indeed emerges a Zen consciousness of each art/act as a sacred act, containing the entire universe of caring–healing practices. Within the modern version of nursing, consider bedmaking and handwashing, which were considered nursing fundamentals: procedures for both comfort and sanitation. In this Zen consciousness, handwashing still adheres to the cleanliness and germ theory of sanitation for the elimination of contamination but it additionally becomes a symbolic purification act. Handwashing can serve as a form of meditation, a moment to pause, contemplate and center. It can serve as an occasion for clearing one's energy, opening up one's system to be both cleansed and open to receive again. It contains an act of 'purification and self-care' (influenced by Sherri Abbott, doctoral student).

Bedmaking and handwashing are only two examples that can offer new caring occasions for self and other. With an expanded mode of consciousness, take any of the conventional, premodern, modern, to postmodern caring acts—mouth and foot care, the range of motion exercises, touching, administering techniques and medications, feeding, toileting, and assisting with any and all basic human needs. All these acts are subject to a redefinition and reconsideration within the postmodern/transpersonal framework of expanded consciousness. They can be seen again, as if for the first time, as occasions for caring and healing, as art/acts, as sacred acts, as Zen acts, each containing and holding up the entire universe of caring. They return nursing and other healing practitioners to 'reclaiming the body' and embodied caring–healing acts. They are undertaken with an intentional consciousness and awareness that any act serves as a vehicle toward healing, wholeness and integrity.

Within the postmodern/transpersonal framework, nursing arts, skills, or 'fundamentals' remain 'essential', but for entirely different reasons. For once one has an expanded consciousness and a different intentionality, it is no longer appropriate, nor acceptable, to engage in technical, routine, body-physical care, administered as a job 'to get done', as people who need 'to be done', as techniques to be mechanically and technically completed to persons as bodies. Something new has to transpire in the practitioner if he or she is to engage in the Zen of caring.

Nursing, individually and collectively, becomes part of the ontological shift necessary for demonstrating the so-called Zen awareness. Any and all caring–healing acts can serve as sacred or profane acts. Even though the nurse may not carry out all the 'fundamentals', it is nursing as a professional entity which holds and carries the consciousness of caring for the whole—the sacred feminine. It is nursing's caring consciousness, Zen consciousness, which provides the oversight of caring and healing within the universe of caring in the system.

This is why nursing administrators and advanced clinical practitioners become so important in determining and sustaining the nature of caring–healing within a given system. The nurse is the one who helps to hold, disseminate and administer the caring–healing consciousness of the whole in each single object and act, knowing that each single act points toward all other practices for an individual, system or community. The Zen of caring, contained in each act, within a new consciousness of the whole, becomes a new healing ethic for both nursing and health care systems for the new millennium.

Transpersonal nursing as ontological *architect*

16

Caring–healing architecture within the postmodern/ transpersonal paradigm

As we move into the postmodern/transpersonal model, we awaken to the fact that we breathe in our surroundings with all of our senses. We recognize that an architectural environment that is faceless, harsh and sterile can actually make us feel unwell, exhausted and disconnected with ourselves and our energy source, thus contributing to a lack of connectedness and lack of community. Day (1990) pointed out that some modern architecture, especially hospitals, can actually be abusive to people, the environment and nature. The predominant theme in modern architecture is one that promotes straight lines and forms, spaces, shapes, lines and colors that are decontextualized, disconnecting us from the relationships between the elements. This modern style is in sharp contrast to premodern harmony of nature, form and shape as depicted in the healing sanctuary (e.g. Sanctuario de Chimayo in Chimayo, New Mexico, USA, Fig. 16.1, an example of premodern healing space).

Day said that the anonymity of modern architecture and environment can be 'life sapping'. Modern architecture was seen as an objective physical space created to contain bodies, one might say a 'warehouse for bodies' (Fig. 16.2). In another sense, it has been explained this way:

Postmodernism is perhaps too comforting a term. It tells you what you are leaving (spare, little boxes, tight little concepts) without committing you to any particular

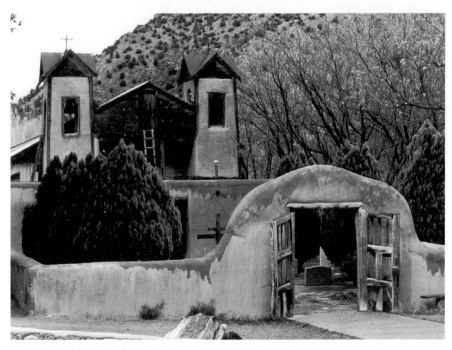

Figure 16.1 Premodern architecture: traditional healing space. (Sanctuario de Chimayo, New Mexico, USA. Photograph by Dr Rose S Le Roux 1987. Reproduced with permission.)

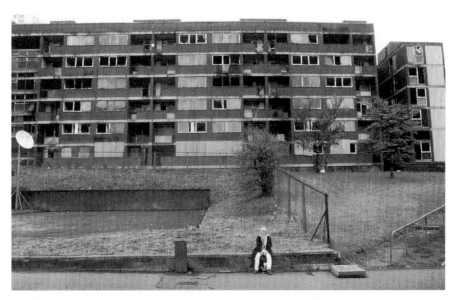

Figure 16.2 Modern architecture: 'a warehouse for bodies'. (Glasgow, Scotland, UK. Reproduced with permission of Dr Philip Darbyshire.)

destination … it conveys the impression that modernism is over—but in fact we
still haven't emerged from the spare, little, tight boxes and concepts,—[we are] still
busy doing nothing more than working changes on the same tight, little concepts
for the benefit of one another.   (Janck 1987, in: Wolfe 1987, p.130)

The concepts of modern and postmodern have their origin in architecture. Toulmin (1990) observed that the beginning of the end of modernity
was reflected most dramatically in the work of the American architect
Venturi who argued that the age of the modern had passed and that architecture must now yield to a new postmodern style. This style reintroduced
elements of beauty, local color, decoration, historical references and even
playfulness and fantasy (Fig. 16.3). It sought the ascendancy of beauty,
connection and wholeness over strict lines and straight lines per se, using
as examples, the extremes from featureless, block institutions that served
as isolated suburban houses, hospitals and military bases and public
offices. Some of the postmodern styles sought harmony and offered an
almost frivolous alternative to the institutional darkness and starkness of
the modern architectural period.

This approach can be seen in Scotland, in the modern-style architecture
of Glasgow architect–engineer Charles Rennie Mackintosh. His famous
Hill House stands as a work of esthetic art, with minimalist beauty and
lines, which were later taken to an extreme by others within the modernist
style. Mackintosh would not have approved of the inappropriate extension
of his work that resulted in stark housing projects now in existence outside
Glasgow and other cities worldwide, projects providing disconnected,
lonely, ugly places for bodies but with no place for the soul. They remain
separated from social, natural and cultural meaning, and also from the
everyday life of the people who dwell there. To quote Wolfe (1987):

The 'modern' architectural movement was captured by the postwar school which
opened in Weimar, Germany in 1919, under the direction of architect Walter
Gropius. Even then, the famous Bauhaus school became a radical approach to art
in all its forms—a philosophical center. Its distinctive chant was 'starting from

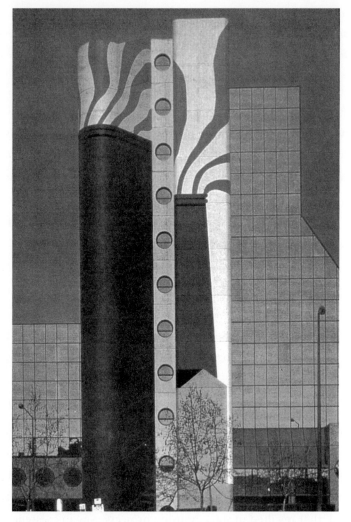

Figure 16.3 Postmodern architecture: 'a search for beauty, evolving new forms beyond the modern'. (National Tax Building, Lisbon, Portugal 1978. From 'Tomas Taveira' 1991. © Academy Editions/Tomas Taveira. Reprinted with permission.)

zero'—wiping out connections, continuity, context relation—all those notions so now desperately called for within the postmodern.

These features of modern architecture and the idea of 'starting from zero' were so sterile that members of the school had to keep adding garlic to their food in order for it to have any taste, because it too was bland and pure like the Bauhaus style. What resulted became the squat, concrete blockhouses, dust and blasted skyscrapers which disfigure our lives and now have to be 'redesigned with postmodern flair.

As Dostoevsky suggested, ideas have consequences. Toulmin emphasized that modernity as a worldview started long before the 1890 era of Mackintosh and could be traced back to Kant's and Descartes' logic and epistemology of rationality. He reminded us that, despite all the ambiguities surrounding the idea of modernity—the varied dates, people and disciplines—and whether defects lie with architecture, science, the worldview, or with modern technology, 'all parties to the debate agree that the modern world committed us to thinking about nature, humans and institutions in a new and scientific way and to using more rational methods to deal with the problems of human life and society' (Toulmin 1990, p. 9). This perspective, of course, extended directly into the modern medicine revolution, which reached its pinnacle in the 20th century. In general, modern modes of thought and practices were reset on a rational approach to life and became the foundation for all serious fields of intellectual inquiry—nursing notwithstanding!

Straight lines and rectangular forms are not forms found anywhere in the human body, in human movement, human activity, nor anywhere in nature. Rectangular forms and straight lines suit machines and mechanistic thinking. Things that are alive never fit into a hard-edged category. A world made up of rectangles is death to the soul. Hard-minded matter, hard lines, hard corners and repetitive, unambiguous forms dehumanize space.

Tom Wolfe described the Bauhaus school as a movement which enshrined geometric solids, cubes and cylinders; it chose the most economical form for a machine age. We now need public and private spaces which are spirit nourishing, spatial and sensory—buildings whose architectural qualities are infused with the colors of human life. As Wolfe (1987) put it, nothing contributes so much to social (and spiritual) malaise as the anonymity of modern architecture: the feeling that you know no one, and no one cares.

The consequences of the architectural movements have manifested themselves in our hospitals and public institutions where we attempt to undertake our caring–healing practices. They reinforce the view that people can be controlled and altered by the spaces in which they live and work, resulting in a 'policing of the impulses' and the human condition of those who live and work in sterile, anemic surroundings (Wolfe 1987, p. 15). The current attempt to redesign hospitals and recreate esthetic, even home-like, space is a response to the views of the people who reside and work there, as well as to the views of patients, families, visitors and loved ones. Such efforts have improved the overall image of hospitals within the community and among the public. While helpful, the systems still fall short as healing spaces.

As noted by my colleague Dr Alice Davidson, a nurse expert in healing space and the environment, these efforts at redesign still reside within a 'hospitality model' (Davidson, personal communication, 1992). Such models are evident in hotels and airports. To make the turn to post-modern/transpersonal, a more radical shift is required: one that attends to healing within an expanded consciousness model, promoting the intentional healing role of architecture alongside conscious, intentional, caring–healing modalities.

A conscious attention to healing space shifts a hospital from being simply a place for bodies to be controlled, manipulated, treated and then turned loose. Even though a patient may receive the finest of modern medical–technical approaches to cure in the most advanced architecturally designed hospital units, no healing can occur without some conscious awareness and promotion of wholeness—an attention to body, mind and spirit as one.

Jain Malkin (1992) suggested that the new frontier for health care design would be the creation of healing environments designed to attend to the relationship between stress and illness and to hospital stress factors. On a deeper level, new developments are focusing on the senses. The latest research in PNI makes explicit the relationship between emotions and immunological dysfunctions, and the ability of the senses (hearing, sight, smell, touch and taste) to influence emotions, for better or for worse (Malkin 1992).

Within this new/old way of understanding the environment, basic attention is once again being given, or needs to be given, to environmental essentials. This would involve, for example, noise reduction, and the intentional introduction of art, music and mythology as expressions of humanity and culture. These aspects of the environment touch the deepest core of our being and can assist in transcending illness, pain and suffering, helping us to remember our common humanity.

Other environmental dimensions include conscious actions upon the chakras through the use of color therapy and what Gerber (1988) calls 'vibrational medicine', where each visible color of the chakra system is aligned with the particular energy center. An understanding of the energetic links of color to body physiology within the chakra centers is just beginning to be discovered in Western medicine.

Another aspect of a healing environment that is being incorporated into new systems of healing is smell, and the influence of aromatherapy. The associations of medicinal smells within hospitals produce a negative emotion and anxiety. Unpleasant odors are known to increase heart rate and respiration, while pleasant fragrances lower blood pressure and heart rate (Malkin 1992, p. 20).

Within this line of thinking about healing architecture, much needs to be learned about the life-enhancing possibilities of architecture and the creation of healing spaces. Many of these dimensions overlap with the caring–healing modalities that nurses and other health professions can control and alter, even before the architecture is changed.

Nevertheless, we are now seeing an increased awareness of the importance of healing space, based upon Rudolf Steiner's early theory of anthroposophy (science of the spirit). Steiner (1861–1925) was an Austrian-born scholar, scientist and artist. His goal was to engage the person in the conscious process of self-healing and spiritual growth, seeing illness as an opportunity for transformation and/or evolving consciousness. Anthroposophic architecture such as Steiner's makes intentional use of organic shapes, color, textures, lighting and views of nature to consciously enhance healing. Along with the architecture, as seen in Figure 16.4 (an anthroposophically designed healing temple concept in Europe), specific therapies—such as mineral baths, massage, music, sculpture and painting—are used to consciously and intentionally restore harmony and equilibrium.

This aspect of healing architecture and healing space seeks to unify opposites and honor indigenous native healing beliefs, such as 'nature as healer'. This progressive line of thinking seeks to incorporate the therapeutic potential into all aspects of the environment, including the consciousness of practitioners.

Malkin (1992, pp. 36–37) has developed a guide to creating a healing environment which intentionally aims to enhance immunity, and which is complementary to the effects of drugs and medical technology. It seeks to reduce the length of hospital stay (and consequently the cost), and create a greater sense of harmony, healing and positive outcomes with an illness or hospital experience. The factors Malkin suggests should be considered in a healing environment are depicted in Box 16.1.

In reconsidering Nightingale's *Notes on Nursing* (1992 commemorative edition) explicit references were made to the environment's effects on health and healing. During the latter part of the 20th century, see how relevant the environment now is. It was not so long ago, for example, that we scoffed at the notion of bottled water; now its use is mainstream, out of necessity. With our polluted cities and contaminated air, the pursuit

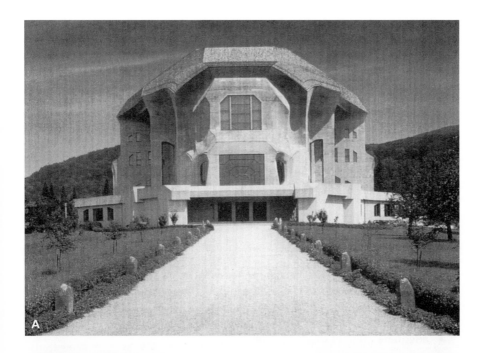

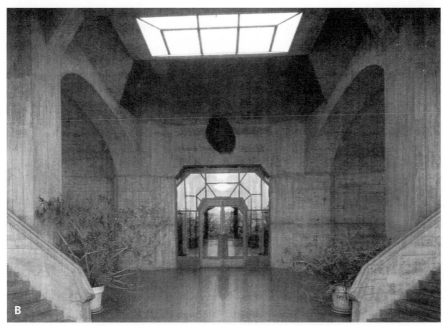

Figure 16.4 'Healing temple' architecture in Europe: (A) front view exterior, (B) interior, west staircase. (From 'Rudolph Steiner, Goetheanum, Dornach' by Wolfgang Pehnt. Photographs by Thomas Dix, © 1991. Reprinted with permission.)

Box 16.1 Developing a healing environment. (From 'Hospital Interior Architecture' by J Malkin © 1992. Reprinted with permission of John Wiley & Sons, Inc., New York.)

Many factors have to be considered in the creation of a healing environment:

1 *Noise control*
- sound of footsteps in corridor
- slamming doors, clanking latches
- loudspeaker paging system
- staff conversations from nurse stations or staff lounge
- other patients' televisions and radios
- clanking of dishes on food carts.

2 *Air quality*
- need for fresh air, solarium or roof garden
- avoidance of noxious off-gassing from synthetic materials, including certain types of paint
- avoidance of odiferous cleaning agents
- adequate number of air changes.

3 *Thermal comfort*
- ability to control room temperature, humidity and air circulation to suit personal needs.

4 *Privacy*
- ability to control view of the outdoors
- ability to control social interaction and view of patient in adjacent bed
- secure place for personal belongings
- place to display personal mementos (family photos, get-well cards, flowers).

5 *Light*
- non-glare lighting in patient room
- ability to control intensity of light
- good reading light
- window should be low enough for patient to see outdoors while lying in bed
- lighting in patient's room should be full spectrum.

6 *Communication*
- ability to contact staff when needed
- comfortable places to visit with family
- television, radio and telephone available as needed.

7 *Views of nature*
- views of trees, flowers, mountains or ocean from patient's rooms and lounges
- indoor landscaping.

8 *Color*
- careful use of color to create mood, lift spirit, and make rooms cheerful
- use in bedlinens, bedspreads, gowns, personal hygiene kits, accessories, food trays.

9 *Texture*
- introduction of textural variety in wall surfaces, floors, ceilings, furniture, fabrics and artwork.

10 *Accommodation for families*
- provide place for family members to make them feel welcome, rather than intrusive
- provide visitor lounges and access to vending machines, telephones, and cafeteria.

of clear air is now a worldwide priority. Even at a precursory level, Nightingale remarked on the environmental categories of noise, sound, light, air, taste, sanitation, water, cleanliness, esthetics–beauty, variety, views, pets, trees, nature, children, music, color, form, flowers, paintings, proper nutrition, bed and sleep. These are all non-invasive, non-intrusive, natural modalities that have their own significance and importance in one's healing.

Whether in a modern or postmodern paradigm, nursing still has a long way to go in attending to the environment and the basic caring arts, as instructed by the Nightingale tradition. Nursing and other health professionals in the future, whether working in a hospital or creating new centers for caring–healing, will need to be involved in at least two missions:

- creating caring–healing spaces, environmentally and transpersonally
- being a part of healing relationships, systems, and communities.

Within the postmodern/transpersonal model, we move to consider architecture as creating space and a place for humans to live and expand their awareness and consciousness; to consciously and intentionally create architecture that Christopher Day (1990) framed as 'places of the soul'. Transpersonal architecture within the postmodern caring–healing perspective becomes akin to psychoarchitecture/sacred geometry—spiritual architecture which provides a natural environment with beauty, art, nature, trees, waterfalls, flowers, natural light and color. Transpersonal architecture draws upon myth, symbol, metaphor, ancient form and archetype to tap into our common humanity for individual and collective healing; this type of architecture helps us connect and remember ourselves as *one*.

In a transpersonal healing space, music and sound, for example, will be selected more for their physics and soothing–healing power than for what might be considered the traditional appeal of composer, style and selection (although that is still integrated into individual options). Some of these views of healing architecture have been presented by Kaiser and others (unpublished paper, 1988) in creating 'hospitals for the 21st century.' These hospitals will not, of course, be 'hospitals' at all, in the modern sense of the word. They will more nearly be caring–healing centers with spa-like conditions, designed to appeal to evolving consciousness, to the care of mindbodyspirit and to all bodily senses as embodied spirit. They will address what we now consider to be the 'care of the soul.'

Symbolic and sacred archetypal architecture becomes a part of post-modern healing spaces; the mythological, archetypal symbolism becomes a means by which one can tap into inner healing, to facilitate one in reconnecting and remembering one's humanity—tapping into the collective humanity, the sacred unconscious, to reunite with other cultures, and experience diverse yet shared meanings of humanity across cultures. The effect helps to restore greater harmony and wholeness to all who work within this space. Such architecture resonates with the human soul, since myths, archetypes, beauty and nature transcend the whole being across time and conditions.

Kaiser (unpublished paper, 1988) suggests that doctors, nurses and hospital administrators are actually mythmakers. Just as modern medical science told one story about life, illness, disease, health, healing and caring (usually stories about body disease and treatment rather than other aspects of healing), the next era is charged with transforming the mythic, sterile hospital of the late 20th century. Conventional, functional architecture will be transformed into a system of healing and caring, bestowing and conferring new meaning for person, family and community with respect to environment and healing space. Nursing has a major role to play in making meaning for the old/new mythic institutions of healing. Healing myths are already embedded in nursing's archetypal lines across the history of the sacred feminine and women as healers. During the modern era, healing rituals, myths and metaphors were all but excluded from the institutions; indeed, they were all but excluded from nursing's consciousness, in spite of Nightingale's astute advice of over 100 years ago.

Part of the emerging postmodern/transpersonal awareness in nursing is in creating new possibilities, and making explicit in consciousness the intentionality that caring arts can potentiate wholeness. Likewise, the lack of this perspective in our practices and our institutions can actually deform the human experience and obstruct healing. The environment, in this instance, takes on an ontological design aspect to parallel the ontological competencies of the health professionals. Within an ontological design framework for architecture and healing environments, the soulful needs of human(s) need to be attended to, acknowledging the need for healing, wholeness, authenticity, relationship, consciousness and intentionality. The intentionality and consciousness do not mean that the nurse abandons the medical regime skills and practices. Rather, it means that the background now becomes reintegrated, reinterpreted, redefined and requestioned with respect to the caring–healing context and consciousness.

Perhaps this is where we might also consider the philosophical, rhetorical idea, that with every physical condition, there is a metaphysical mirror. The model of ontological design for caring acts and healing space now has to be reconsidered, to determine if it can accommodate the integration of the physical and metaphysical, mythical, metaphorical, symbolic and archetypal aspects of healing. It is not just a matter of 'fixing things' or trying to cure the body physical ailment.

Regardless of one's disciplinary background or practice role in the system, all health professionals in this model will need to be ontologically and technologically competent. They will need to know how to mediate between those two critical junctures, both of which are now becoming a sine qua non for the new millennium.

The tranquilized environment of modern hospitals now calls for an awareness and an awakening, and for the need to make explicit another emerging paradigm beyond the archaic body treatment, beyond the technology-and-cure dominance. One of the requirements of postmodern/transpersonal health professionals and educators is to help us all to 'see' this new model of possibilities, the range of new meanings and the role of mythical and archetypal features that appeal to the soul. They need to help us access the essential features of the experience and help us reinterpret healing to the public. This change is transformative for all involved in health care.

Kaiser (unpublished paper, 1988) has remarked that sick hospitals cannot heal patients; now we have to pay attention to the subtle environment of the hospital. Kaiser reminds us that a highly negative worker can contaminate the mental and spiritual ambiance of the entire institution, including the patient's room. This line of thinking is consistent with Zukav's (1990) thesis on light and energy (that lower-frequency feelings will drain energy from higher-frequency feelings).

Nurses are often experts in controlling the subtle environment, and they have almost total control over a patient's environment. In spite of

Nightingale's attention to environment, and in spite of the nursing meta-paradigm including environment as part of its subject matter and practice focus, nursing has not systematically heeded this domain in practice.

Nurses as ontological architects

Within postmodern/transpersonal nursing, nurses will need to play a critical role in creating healing space, facilitating, if not creating and directing, ontological design projects whereby professionals, employees, patients, friends, family, volunteers, visitors, community members and any members of the public who enter the space will experience a transforming, regenerating, healing environment (influenced by Kaiser).

Kaiser (unpublished paper, 1988) describes such space as providing experiences with nature—a natural environment. It might be a space where selected music anoints you as you walk through open corridors, and where symbolic architecture with archetypal, mythological images, perhaps stained glass windows, await you. Medical technology and medical personnel are unobtrusive. Light, color, texture and sound are highlighted.

This kind of postmodern psychoarchitecture is designed to potentiate an evolving consciousness. It is designed to alter consciousness and can be employed to stimulate and facilitate transpersonal transcendental experience. As Kaiser explains, 'wall murals, pictures and the statuary will need to resonate with the ancient myths and sacred archetypes of humankind'.

Kaiser concludes that 'the future hospital does not look like, sound like, smell like, feel like, or taste like the hospitals of our [modern] era'. Consistent with the ontological competencies and caring–healing modalities for nursing, nurses within the postmodern/transpersonal frame will need to be ontological architects, creating healing space and providing ontologically based healing modalities of care.

The postmodern/transpersonal nurse creates, shapes and 'holds' space for healing. The nurse within this consciousness deals with both the non-physical and the physical environment, and with the manifest and the subtle environment, including the energy, mood and ambiance of the setting. The notion of ontological architect brings a whole new meaning to Nightingale's advice that the nurse's role is 'to put the patient in the best condition where nature can heal' (1992 commemorative edition).

The nurse and all health practitioners are now challenged to coordinate, mediate and work collaboratively with a full range of modalities and practitioners in addition to:

- the nurse's ontological presence through a caring–healing consciousness
- the nurse creating space for healing
- the nurse engaging in artistry through ontological caring–healing practices.

Kaiser (unpublished paper, 1988) predicted that the hospital of the future would have over 40 experiences available to patients; music, massage, relaxation, visualization, educational videotapes, humor, friendly visitation, pet therapy, prayer groups, healing touch, lifework counseling and biofeedback are only a few of the modalities he envisioned. Such a model for the postmodern era will also embrace technology such as informatics and virtual realities. Healing modalities which help patients to repattern and alter consciousness will be made available for the purposes of spiritual emergence and transformative integration. The nurse may become an expert in one or a range of these modalities, but he or she is also challenged to revision the way in which traditional nursing arts can be redefined as part of any system of care.

Part of the role of ontological architect includes a reconsideration of symbol and ritual, so much a part of nursing's roots. Recreating meaningful ritual is one way in which the nurse can shape space to activate and potentiate a person's natural healing system. The postmodern/ transpersonal nurse truly becomes a sacred architect.

The hospital of the future, within the postmodern/transpersonal model, will need to create a sacred space. In this sacred space, illness becomes a special opportunity for someone to become more aware of, and to be authentically empowered at, the soul energy level. In this new space, one can experience consciousness-altering architecture and processes that help to repattern and/or potentiate wholeness, healing, self-knowledge, self-control, and self-healing possibilities.

This thinking is what Moore (1992) referred to as 'honoring symptoms as a voice of the soul'. In this framework, the environment would reflect the cosmological relationship between human and the universe (McKahan, unpublished paper, 1988). Rituals and acts of caring become critical dimensions of such a paradigm proposed for the future.

These activities and this line of thinking are all consistent with Nightingale's original writings, but are taken forward into the trans- personal dimension. In considering transpersonal healing space there is the need to recreate meaningful ritual as part of the caring–healing practices evoking art, beauty and soul care.

17

Unconcluding postmodern Nightingale[1]

....

Would you do nothing then, in cholera, fever ...?

....

... so deep-rooted and universal is the conviction that to give medicine is to be doing something, or rather everything: to give air, warmth, cleanliness ... is to do nothing ... The very elements of ... nursing are ... little understood.

(Nightingale, 1992 commemorative edition, p. 6)

From one century to another, from one turn-of-the-century to another, Florence Nightingale's vision and wisdom ring true and speak to us still. Through the ages, her voice can be heard more loudly than ever, if we listen, if we are ready to hear the calling, if we are ready to consider anew her timeless message in this era.

Her century-old thinking about nursing proclaimed and foreshadowed the emerging caring, sacred, feminine energy consciousness still awakening in our time. Nightingale's proclamation was a call to women and men and to nursing consciousness as the repository of both knowledge and wisdom, a significant social, political, and humane force in overcoming ignorance toward basic health, human caring and healing.

---

[1]From Watson 1992b, pp. 80–85, © Lippincott Williams & Wilkins, Philadelphia. Reproduced with permission.

This health knowledge and wisdom, so desperately needed in her time, remains the call and manifesto of our time. It is the need to:

- reiterate the interconnection between person and environment, between person and nature, between the inner and outer worlds, between the private and the public, between the physical and the spiritual as part of the natural healing responses of people and civilizations
- systematically develop nursing, even if by another name
- have a developed nursing service where people are cared for by qualified nurses
- ensure nurses do not have to forfeit a proper education
- enhance the quality of nursing and human caring, healing and health services offered to the public.

Even though the roots of nursing throughout time have been based on a philosophy of and commitment to caring and healing, and on all the insights from Nightingale, ironically we find ourselves at the end of the 20th century, a century of revolution in biomedical science, having to return to the ancient vision of Nightingale to make a case for basic human caring–healing, health knowledge and practices. Indeed, nursing has yet to fulfill the promise of Nightingale's vision as a mature health profession:

> It is extraordinary that, whereas the laws of the motions of the heavenly bodies, far removed as they are from us, are perfectly well understood, the laws of the human mind, which are under our observation all day, every day, are no better understood now than they were 2000 years ago. But how much more extraordinary is it that ... neither mothers (fathers, sic) ... nor nurses of hospitals are taught anything about those laws which God has assigned to the relations of our bodies with the world in which He has put them.
>
> (1992 commemorative edition, p. 7)

Nightingale's view of the need for knowledge of the human mind is akin to the latest developments in this time related to the roles of consciousness and intentionality and new views of the body. Her insights coincide with the latest developments in mind–body medicine—all necessary in understanding the connections between the basic laws of the universe and the world of inner healing.

Just as a century ago nursing was considered to be a 'calling', there is once again an open call for compassion, commitment and involvement—a passion, if you will, for nurses to recommit themselves to a calling to engage in reform based on basic human caring–healing and health values. This reform is based on knowledge rooted in ancient feminine wisdom, a cosmology of wholeness, connectedness and harmony that needs to once again be openly pronounced for personal, public, scientific and political action.

Nightingale's attunement to the interconnections between and among all dimensions of the personal, the public, and the political parallels the voice of contemporary women who remind us again, in postmodern terms, that the personal *is* the political. The feminist energy voice of this era takes on deeper significance when reconsidered within the historical backdrop of Nightingale's strong message to make the private work and world of women's (caring–healing) knowledge and wisdom a source of public and political importance. This private, ancient feminine wisdom of healing, once brought to the public and political consciousness, can become the foundation for societal and system reform and transformation.

This ancient Nightingale wisdom is also part of nursing's theories of caring. The 'carative factors' in my first book, *Nursing. The Philosophy and Science of Caring* (Watson 1979), are highly consistent with Nightingale's call for a values-based approach to the nursing profession and a oneness of mindbodyspirit with respect to caring needs. We share a concern for the humanistic, the altruistic, the spiritual, the scientific, the existential, but also a concern for basic caring practices, the nursing arts, as well as 'the health of houses' (and now communities). This shared thinking seeks to recognize and restore the connections between person–environment–nature and the connection between the physical and metaphysical. It also seeks to recognize and restore the relationship between health and wholeness, with respect to such factors as noise, light, air, color, touch and a variety of stimuli.

Nightingale's philosophy of spiritual consciousness is consistent with contemporary and ancient principles of yoga, meditation and imagery practices. These spiritual practices can and are being used in both religious and secular settings—settings which are increasingly integrating such practices into health care as forms of caring–healing arts (Macrae 1995).

Caring practices that emerge from my carative factors and from new dimensions of transpersonal caring and healing attend to feelings, relationships, teaching–learning, caring moments, context, consciousness and concrete actions related to a supportive, protective, or corrective mental, physical, sociocultural and spiritual environment. Variables affecting external and internal environments such as stress, change, comfort needs, privacy and clean–aesthetic surroundings are all carative factors that are very Nightingale in their approach.

This pervasive aspect of nursing, transmitted by Nightingale's writings as well as by contemporary caring work, requires that the caring knowledge of women and nurses no longer remains hidden. Nursing's work today again requires strong voices, a being-in-the-world, courageously and convincingly conveying a new proclamation for reform in the personal, public, political and social thinking and acting of our time.

Caring writing today shares a century-old national and global agenda with Nightingale. We continue to be informed and inspired by the rich, often hidden, ordinary caring–healing knowing of nursing and women. This so-called ordinary knowing advocated by Nightingale was also valued as extraordinary. Ordinary knowing becomes extraordinary when we enter into human caring with a spiritual sense of awe and reverence, with a sense of the fantastic. This kind of calling provides us with the clear values essential to sustaining compassion, commitment and caring in instances where people and society are threatened, biologically or otherwise. The ordinary caring, taken for granted in nursing, transforms into the extraordinary to inform our vision, our way of seeing and our way of being, knowing and doing as asserted by Nightingale.

Some of Nightingale's seeing and knowing included ancient insights and values that parallel current human caring theory. This theory is based on caring as a moral ideal and aims to guide nursing education, praxis and clinical inquiry. It allows for the spiritual, the transcendent and the whole, while attending to fully embodied being and doing. Some of Nightingale's seeing and knowing included a vision and image of completeness, of beauty and harmony of life, a sense of oneness with all living things.

Some of this timeless Nightingale seeing and knowing is congruent with the emerging caring–healing paradigm of our time that speaks of the natural healing processes, the inner healer and the need for being connected with nature. All of this timeless seeing and knowing presented by Nightingale, a woman of vision, remains. Elsewhere, it is reflected in contemporary human-caring nursing theory; but this so-called extraordinary seeing and knowing is yet to totally emerge in nursing.

Just as Nightingale's (1859) *Notes on Nursing* said that the very elements of nursing were all but unknown, so is this true over a century later. One of the messages of nursing caring theory today is a call for the restoration of basic values, commitment and informed moral action that leads to social and political action. Nursing caring theory continues to reiterate a call for the search for new caring knowledge and caring praxis: practice informed by human values and an ethos of caring. This unknown knowledge requires a continuing search for new relationships between elements of human caring and healing processes and health experiences. Although Nightingale's caring–healing model has transcended time and is prophetic for this century's health reform, the model is yet truly to come of age in nursing and the health care system. Nightingale's enduring voice remains before us as a part of pressing public, political, and scientific agendas, in spite of our politically and scientifically renowned turn-of-the-century institutions.

Nightingale's enduring public health and human caring proclamations

Is all this premature suffering and death necessary?

(1992 commemorative edition)

If we reconsider Nightingale in the light of a general philosophy and theory of caring, her voice parallels the public and political consciousness of today. It is timely to pronounce once again the human significance of basic public health and human caring within the Nightingale model. Today, the AIDS epidemic and reports of malaria, measles and cholera outbreaks around the world are reminiscent of the situation in Nightingale's time. Just as in the 1800s, the call today is still for the reform of basic human caring and health practices with respect to the homeless, the medically indigent, those who are HIV positive or living with AIDS or other incurable or chronic illness, and those who are often neglected, such as pregnant women, children and elderly people.

Calls for health care and system reform are just as prevalent worldwide today as they were then. These calls are in the form of personal, social and political action. With the blight of the American health care (read 'sick care') system, there are now requests to create 'dedicated caring–healing units' and practices in and out of our institutions. There are calls to deal with the epidemic of diseases caused by social, political and scientific neglect; calls to counterbalance technologic imperatives; calls to attend to basic human comfort measures, such as human touch, massage, relaxation and mood changes. There are social and political action calls to attend to the quality of living and dying; calls to encompass natural and aesthetic surroundings that attend to light, form, air, color and nature; calls to be equally concerned with and present to the spiritual/metaphysical elements of caring–healing; calls to be concerned with relationships and unity and wholeness; calls to be concerned with consciousness and the transcendence of self with respect to higher self and one's own inner healer. The contexts for all these approaches are basic public health issues that are humanitarian as well as scientific and political. Nightingale's earlier thinking calls for a very similar caring–healing model today as part of a mandate for health reform.

Post-postmodern messages from Nightingale

Just as at the turn of the past century, we once again need social and political action based on a worldview and metaparadigm that has roots in women's sacred wisdom and knowledge. This knowledge can be a basis for a profession, but it is also wisdom beyond knowledge that can be transmitted. The writings of Nightingale remain contemporary and timeless. We can now reconsider the timeless themes, themes that are a part of our awakening, our emerging with a sacred feminine consciousness as part of the social rebalancing called for as the next century greets us.

In summary, there are several pervasive themes from Nightingale and her time that mirror basic philosophy and theories of human caring in contemporary nursing and health care. They are the:

- restoration of basic nursing caring–healing practices
- reintegration of the moral, the spiritual and the metaphysical
- emergence of women's knowledge and values, the sacred feminine healing spirit
- return of a sense of a 'calling' to the profession
- public's request for personal and professional caring competencies and commitments

- honoring of the wisdom of connected oneness and wholeness; the interrelationship between and among person–nature–environment/ caring–healing and health
- recognition of the interrelationship between and among the personal, the political, the social, the scientific and the spiritual.

Nightingale's insight and worldview hold power and vision for these postmodern/transpersonal times in nursing's history, just as they did in her own time. Her voice still offers prescient recommendations for health care reform that is called for now as loudly as in 1859, when *Notes on Nursing* was written. This reform speaks largely to women, but also to men and to the public, about the personal health care and health knowledge required by everyone.

Nightingale's views on nursing, her vision, commitment and dedication to nursing and nurses, continue to be foundational, informative and inspirational, if not prophetic. Caring–healing health reform in nursing builds on what we now know as a sacred feminine cosmology. Nursing can enter the future with authentic connections for both moral and political inspiration and action. Perhaps this time, a century later, a postmodern/ transpersonal, sacred-conscious nursing will finally reclaim its heritage. Nursing will emerge as the health, human caring, and healing profession for the new millennium.

Are we listening? Do we hear the calling? Are we ready?

18

Relighting the lamp

· ·

If there is light in the soul,
There will be beauty in the person.
If there is beauty in the person,
There will be harmony in the house.
If there is harmony in the house,
There will be order in the nation.
If there is order in the nation,
There will be peace in the world.   (Chinese proverb)

There is a relationship between caring and peace in our personal lives and caring and peace in our world. Light and ritual are both metaphors and symbols for nursing to imagine another way, beyond the modern, of how things might be. It is ritual and light which can create a path to reconnect nursing with its past–present–future. If any one image pervades nursing's history, it is the light of Nightingale's lamp, radiating the meaning of nursing's light and energy to the world.

Postmodern/transpersonal nursing is about 'relighting the metaphorical lamp' (Bradshaw 1996) and helping nursing to reintegrate, reconnect and provide continuity to its own wholeness, wholeness that has been wounded during nursing's modern era.

Rituals become an outer form of myth; they are acts that are repeated as archetypal actions across time. Fox (1991) believes that we need a revolution in ritual. Barry Lopez, the naturalist, said one element of myth (and ritual) is to separate the authentic from the inauthentic (1989). The power of both is to nurture, heal and repair a spirit of disarray. When myth and ritual are integrated, we use story power to reorder a state of chaos and confusion by contact with some pervasive, archetypal truths. Art and architecture, along with myth, ritual, metaphor and symbol, can all be invocations, opportunities to 'recreate' order and harmony and select enduring relationships with our interior and exterior landscapes (Lopez 1989).

One learns a landscape not by knowing the name or identity of everything in it but by perceiving the relationships in it, by grasping the whole. It is through this tacit knowledge that we engage in a quality of consciousness transformation brought about by the art, ritual, myth, metaphor and symbol. Steven (1953) wrote of the 'symbolic language of "metamorphosis"', reminding us of the relationship between metaphor and metamorphosis, both involving a transformation in the world of consciousness, of meaning.

As Merleau-Ponty (1962, p. xix) and Dillard (1982) reminded us: 'God help us, we are all condemned to meaning'. Meaning is the rock, the foundation—the rock is all there is, in Dillard's sense. Yet this meaning from myth, ritual and metaphor is precisely what brings forth the mystery, expressed in universal themes to help us understand our world. These themes become guides toward the light of our being, from birth to death, through the passage of time, and through the journey of this life, and those past or future.

More specifically, rituals are how people have always passed on their value system to the young, the next generation. During the modern era, nursing became isolated from its rituals and values; yet it is through ritual that a community heals and enlightens itself. It is ritual that brings forth opportunities to celebrate and release—to let go of the modern sterility and disconnection. Light and ritual are used by individuals and groups to celebrate, heal, remember and reconnect with their members and their meanings.

Light is one of the privileged metaphors across premodern and modern times. In premodern time, light was used in the language of mysticism, in religion and by the Greeks and Eastern religions. Ironically, the modern era was considered to be the age of enlightenment, meaning we were rational and had control over our destiny, nature and other living things. It was the age of moving at the speed of light, of the quantum physics language of paradoxical wave and particles of light. It was the age of government, science and the military use of atomic light-energy pinnacles of accomplishment. The enlightenment used energy as light to harness for functional destructive/protective use. The enlightenment was to take us from the primitive dark ages, past and beyond the renaissance, into rational–cognitive awareness.

Perhaps this postmodern Era III/Paradigm III and beyond can best be captured metaphorically as the age of light, which takes us into a new relationship with our being-in-the-world as embodied forms of light, intersecting and coming into our light, metaphorically and evolutionary. We are becoming more god like and divine as we move towards the light of our divinity, a level of connectedness, the oneness of all, attending to the implicate spiritual unfolding and evolving—as the 'lightness of "being"'— wherein the light of the universe is enfolded and embodied into our very existence.

Other plays on this age of light come from developments in quantum physics that suggest matter is condensed as frozen light. Light is the means by which the entire universe enfolds into itself. Light is the fundamental activity in which existence has its ground. Light also represents immediate contact—very high energy. Light is clarity; light illumines; light is energy. Light is love, compassion, understanding and caring. Light can make us whole or heal us.

Light radiates itself as being through particles, 'events' and shadows, through illness, pain and suffering; in shadows, light is revealed. Light radiates itself as life spirit rather than matter; the cleansing wave, the flicker of hope in the night and darkness of the modern era, which is now passing, and which must pass into the *light*.

A candlelight ritual

If there is any one symbol that represents Nightingale and nursing across time, it is a candle and the light that it produces. A candlelight ritual is ingrained in nursing's collective unconscious, but it has been buried, dormant during this modern technological rise. A candlelight ritual of passing and spreading the light represents a periodic regeneration of nursing and the profession of nursing in the best tradition of Florence Nightingale. Such a symbol and myth brings back the best of caring–healing practices to society, allowing the system to use both sides of its brain—honoring the sacred feminine energy along with the balancing of the whole.

A candlelight ritual is both a premodern and a postmodern image that provides integration, continuity and connection for a restoration of what is missing in modern science and technology. It serves as a symbol for 'relighting the lamp' and carrying the light from one century to another. Since 1991, I have consciously and intentionally begun to reintroduce the ritual of candlelight into nursing.

I repeat my personal story here as an invitation to nurses and nursing to heal and transform themselves and the profession, for another era of human history. In doing so, the ritual helps to simultaneously reconnect nursing with its universal truths and archetypal ground of being, so that it becomes more whole, more complete and more mature, letting its light and energy shine into the world.

Personal story

Recreating a meaningful ritual

Recreating meaningful ritual with candlelight began after my Fulbright research and study in Sweden and other Scandinavian countries in 1991. There, in the northern most part of the globe, I became acutely aware of the light/dark cycles of nature in the Arctic Circle where, during the winter months, there is often little more than 1 hour of daylight. This focus on light was mirrored in the midst of daily Swedish life where there was always special attention paid to light and beauty, usually in the form of freshly cut flowers and the frequent use of candles.

What also stood out in my memory was the prominent use of candlelight during most of my talks and lectures. This simple act often transformed the setting and clearly had a role to play in the atmosphere of any seminar, lecture or talk that I delivered.

Thereafter, I began to use candlelight to create a different atmosphere for teaching and learning about caring and healing. For example, upon my return from Sweden, I offered my first national doctoral theory seminar, held over a 4-day period in Colorado. This time, however, I did two things differently. First, I scheduled the seminar outside the sterile institutional, medical setting, instead holding it on the Boulder campus, at the Alumni Center, formerly the residence of the university president. Second, I brought a candle and lit it as background for the setting.

The setting was a large, beauty-filled living-room arrangement, with oriental carpets, fireplace and overstuffed furniture. We arranged the seating in a circle, instead of rows. In doing so, I had almost unconsciously created a very different mood of esthetics, intimacy and relationship; a sense of trust and safety for learning emerged very quickly. The focus of the seminar was on caring theory and caring as an ontology, an ethic and an epistemology, all resulting in a different level of praxis and a different way of being, something that was being experienced in the pedagogy itself.

As the week progressed, without ever mentioning the candle, each student independently went out and bought their own candle. As the class came to a close at the end of the week, the students collectively and spontaneously started creating their own closing 'ritual', using the original candle from the seminar.

Each student lit her or his candle from the original candle, with the expressed purpose of 'honoring their own and each other's light', and of taking the 'light of nursing's caring and healing' back to their colleagues and home institutions and 'passing it on'. This began in January 1992.

After the spontaneous student-generated candlelight ritual of 'passing the light', I followed their lead. Within days of the seminar I was scheduled to travel to New Zealand and Australia. On my journeys, I continued the candlelight ritual with other colleagues, inviting them to reconnect with their light and pass it on.

Since then I have recreated the candlelight ritual with nurses throughout the US and in many countries and settings around the world, inviting nurses to relight the metaphorical lamp, the light of our being, and to transform themselves, returning to their inner and ancient light as a guide to our future.

The ritual

The candlelight ritual begins by telling the story of the cycle of light and dark in Sweden, and continues with an account of the doctoral student seminar candlelight ritual. Then, using what I now call the 'transformer candle', which I carry with me, I recreate the ritual by using it to take light from my original 1992 candle. I then pass on the light, from the original candle, to a new candle which I leave with the group.

The light from the original candle has now been passed around the globe at least twice. There is a passing of the light from the original candle to the newly lit candle, which is left with the sponsoring institution or group. In many instances, even in formal addresses, nurses from the audience have brought their own candles, lighting them from the new one and returning with them to their own setting, to pass on the symbolic light of nursing reawakening, creating points and circles of light throughout the globe. Some who have participated in the candlelight ritual are using their own candles to continue the ritual in their own work, reigniting, regenerating and passing on nursing's caring and healing light in the world. Thousands of nurses around the world are now engaged in and committed to continuing this candlelight ritual. I trust that nurses' and nursing's inner and outer light will continue until we reach a critical mass for the new millennium.

'Holding the light'

The original candle I used in 1992 is now housed in my office at the Center for Human Caring. It is positioned there symbolically as a place that is attempting to hold the light of nursing's caring and healing, and to pass it on to nurses around the world. One of the associates in the UK described her use of the candlelight ritual with nurses at a European nursing conference, and reported that 'the nurses were on their feet applauding, even before the act was completed'.

Nurses and nursing have been cut off from their rituals and archetypal ground of being; nursing has had its light put out, so to speak. When opportunities are offered to reconnect with this level of our being and purpose, a deep level of healing occurs. Nurses talk about 'coming home' to this kind of practice. We are now called upon, wherever we are, to provide space to both metaphorically and literally hold the light and pass it on. All of this evokes what Lewis Mumford (1970) said: 'It is only in a return to our human center, our own light, that transformation can occur'.

The Center for Human Caring and the caring–healing work of nurses and others around the world can join together to recreate meaningful ritual from the light of our center of being. Any and all are invited to participate in passing on the light. For it is through ritual that a community heals itself, ensouls itself, enlightens itself and brings forth opportunities to celebrate and to let go; to begin anew, celebrating a remembering of the light and dark cycles of evolution, change and continuity. The candlelight imprints the archetypal memories of past, present, and future, collecting and gathering them, bringing order to nursing's evolution across time and space.

I recall the Native American saying that every day one should do an act of power and an act of beauty. The act and art of recreating meaningful ritual through relighting the light and passing it on is both an act of power and an act of beauty, calling forth beauty and light into our life and our institutional darkness.

I leave you with the Navajo chant:

'Walk in beauty'—bless the times when inner peace radiates outward, connecting with the order and beauty of nature (the whole).

May you, too, walk in your own power, your own light and your own beauty, and pass it on … radiating caring, healing, and peace to greet the new world.

References

Aberdene P, Naisbitt J 1992 Megatrends for women. Villard Books, New York

Achterberg J 1990 Woman as healer. Shambhala Publications, Boston

Acker K 1997 The Guardian Weekend, London

American Nurses Association 1995 Nursing's social policy statement. American Nurses Publishing, Washington DC, p 6

Ashley J 1976 Hospitals, paternalism and the role of the nursing profession. Teachers' College Press, New York

Bateson M C 1990 Composing a life. Penguin Books, New York

Battista F R 1982 The holographic model, holistic paradigm, information theory and consciousness. In: Wilber K (ed) The holographic paradigm and other paradoxes. New Science Library, Boston, pp 143–149

Beinfield H, Korngold E 1991 Between heaven and earth: a guide to Chinese medicine. Ballantine Books, New York

Benor D 1996 Intention: an experimental focus. Advances in Nursing Science 12(3):4–8

Bingen H 1985 Illuminations of Hildegard of Bingen. (Text by Hildegard of Bingen, commentary by Fox M.) Bear Publications, Santa Fe

Blake W 1796 Auguries of innocence. In: Norton WW 1975 The Norton anthology of poetry, revised. WW Norton, New York, p 555

Bohm D 1986 In: Weber R 1986 Dialogues with scientists and sages: the search for unity. Routledge and Kegan Paul, London

Bohm D 1988 Wholeness and the implicate order. Ark, London

Boulding E 1992 The underside of history, vol 2, rev edn. Sage Publications, Newberry Park, pp 340–341

Bradshaw A 1996 Lighting the lamp: the covenant as an encompassing framework for the spiritual dimension of nursing practice. In: Farmer E (ed) Exploring the spiritual dimension of care. Mark Allen, Quay Books

Briggs J, Peat F D 1989 Turbulent mirror: an illustrated guide to chaos theory and the science of wholeness. Harper & Row, New York

Bronte C 1960 Jane Eyre, 3rd edn. New American Library of World Literature, New York, pp 219, 422–424, 450–451, 459

Buker M 1965 Between man and mind. Macmillan, New York

Byrd R C 1988 Positive therapeutic effects of intercessory prayer in a coronary care unit population. Southern Medical Journal 8:7

Campbell D G 1984 Introduction to the musical brain. MMB Music, St Louis

Campbell D G 1991 The curative potential of sound. In: Campbell D (ed) 1991 Music: physician for time to come. Quest, Wheaton

Campbell (ed) 1992 Music and miracles. Quest, Wheaton

Campbell J 1972 Myths to live by. Viking Press, New York

Coelho P 1993 The alchemist. Harper, San Francisco

Day C 1990 Places of the soul: architecture and environmental design as a healing art. Aquarian Press, London

Denollet J, Sys S U, Stroobant N, Rombouts I I, Gillebert T C, Brutsaert D I 1996 Personality as independent predictor of long-term mortality in patients with coronary heart disease. The Lancet 347:417–421

Department of Health 1992 Health report. HMSO, London

Derrida J 1976 Of grammatology. Johns Hopkins Press, Baltimore

Dillard A 1977 Holy the firm. Harper & Row, New York

Dillard A 1982 Teaching a stone to talk. Harper & Row, New York, p 379

Donoghue D 1983 The arts without mystery. Little Brown, Boston

Dossey B M, Keegan L, Guzzetta C E, Kolkmeier L G 1995 Holistic nursing: a handbook for practice. Aspen, Gaithersburg

Dossey L 1984 Beyond illness. New Science Library, Boulder

Dossey L 1991 Meaning and medicine. Bantam, New York

Dossey L 1993 Healing words, the power of prayer and the practice of medicine. Harper, San Francisco

Dossey L 1996 Distant intentionality: an idea whose time has come. Advances. The Journal of Mind-Body Health 12(3):9–13

Eisler R 1987 The chalice and the blade. Harper, San Francisco

Emerson, R W 1982 Ralph Waldo Emerson selected essays. Penguin American Library, New York, p 48

Epstein G 1996 Mind-body medicine and biological medicine: an unbridgeable gap. Advances 12(3):16–18

Fawcett J 1993 Analysis and evaluation of nursing theories. F A Davis, Philadelphia

Fay F 1987 Critical social theory science. Basil Blackwell Press, Oxford

Fiedler L A 1988 Images of the nurse in fiction and popular culture. In: Jones A (ed) 1988 Images of nursing: perspectives from history, art and literature. University of Pennsylvania Press, Philadelphia, pp 100–112

Foucault M 1984 The means of correct training. In: Rabinow P (ed) The Foucault reader. Pantheon Press, New York

Fox M 1985 (commentary) Illuminations of Hildegard of Bingen. Bear Publications, Santa Fe, p 22

Fox M 1991 Creation spirituality. Harper, San Francisco

Fry S T 1989 Toward a theory of nursing ethics. Advances in Nursing Science 11(4):9–22

Gablik S 1991 The re-enchantment of art. Thames & Hudson, New York

Gadamer H G 1986 The relevance of the beautiful and other essays. Translated by Walker N, Bernasconi R (ed). Cambridge University Press, New York

Gadow S 1988 Covenant without cure: letting go and holding on in chronic illness. In: Watson & Ray M (eds) The ethics of care and the ethics of cure. National League for Nursing, New York, pp 5–14

Gadow S 1994 Whose body? Whose story? Soundings: An Interdisciplinary Journal LXXVII:3–4. Society for Values in Higher Education, Knoxville

Gahrton P 1993 Let grandmothers rule the 2000s: a book about the future.

Gerber R 1988 Vibrational medicine. Bear Publications, Santa Fe

Gilligan C 1982 In a different voice. Harvard University, Cambridge

Greene M 1988 The dialectic of freedom. Teachers College Press, New York

Greene M 1991 Texts and margins. Harvard Educational Review 61(1):25–39

Grey A 1990 Sacred mirrors: the visionary art of Alex Grey. With essays by Wilber K, McCormick C, Grey A. Inner Traditions International, Rochester

Griffin S 1992 A chorus of stones: the private life of war. Doubleday, New York

Griffiths N 1991 Let us think no more of war to end all wars. In: Van de Vanter L, Fuey J A (eds) 1991 Vision of war, dreams of peace. Warner Books, New York, p 201

Hagey R S, McDonough P 1984 The problem of professional labeling. Nursing Outlook 32:151–157

Hall N 1990 The moon and the virgin. In: Murdock M The heroine's journey. Shambhala Publications, Boston

Harman W 1982 The new science and holonomy. In: Wilber K (ed) The holographic paradigm and other paradoxes. New Science Library, Boston, p 139

Harman W 1987a Toward an extended science. Noetic Sciences Review 3:9–14

Harman W 1987b Further comments on an extended science. Commentary. Noetic Sciences Review 4:22–25

Harman W 1991 A reexamination of the metaphysical foundations of modern science. Institute of Noetic Sciences, Sausalito

Harrington L 1988 The diagnosis dilemma: one preferred remedy. Nursing and Health Care 9:93–94

Heidegger M 1971 Poetry, language and thought. Harper & Row, New York

Herbert N 1994 Elemental mind: human consciousness and the new physics. Plume Books, Penguin, New York

Hickson P, Holmes C 1994 Nursing the postmodern body: a touching case. Nursing Inquiry 1:3–14

Hiraki A 1992 Tradition, rationality and power in introductory nursing textbooks: a critical hermeneutics study. Advances in Nursing Science 14(3):1–12

Inner H 1995 New York Times, March 12, p 38

Ironson G, Barr X, Taylor C et al 1992 Effects of anger on left ventricular ejection fraction in coronary artery disease. American Journal of Cardiology 70:281–285

Jackson M 1989 Paths toward a clearing. Radical empiricism and ethnographic inquiry. University of Indiana Press, Bloomington

James W In: Murphy 1992 The future of the body. Explorations into the further evolution of human nature. J P Tarcher, Los Angeles, p 231

Janck C 1987. In: Wolfe T 1987 From Bauchaus to our house. Penguin, London, p 130

Jones A H (ed) 1988 Images of nursing: perspectives from history, art, and literature. University of Pennsylvania Press, Philadelphia

Jung O 1989 In: Tarnas R 1993 The passion of the western mind: understanding the ideas that have shaped our worldview. Ballantine Books, New York

Kalisch B J, Kalisch P A 1982 An analysis of the sources of physician–nurse conflict. In: Muff J (ed) Socialization, sexism and stereotyping: women's issues in nursing. C V Mosby, St Louis, pp 221–233

Kandinsky W 1977 Concerning the spiritual in art. Dover Publications, New York

Kech L R 1995 Sacred eyes. Synergy Associates, Boulder

Keegan L 1996 Healing nutrition. Delmar, Albany, pp 540, 560–561

Keller H 1954 The story of my life. Doubleday, New York

Kim M J, McFarland G K, McLane A M 1991 Pocket guide to nursing diagnoses, 4th edn. Mosby, St Louis

Koerner J G, Bunkers S S 1994. The healing web: an expansion of consciousness. Journal of Holistic Nursing 12(1):51–63

Krieger D 1979 Therapeutic touch. Prentice-Hall, Englewood Cliffs

Krysl M 1980 Poem for the left and right hand. In: More palomino, please, more fuchsia. Cleveland State Poetry Center, Cleveland

Kung H 1982. In: Wilber K (ed) 1982 The holographic paradigm and other paradoxes. New Science, Boston, p4

Lafo R R, Capasso N, Roberts S R 1994 Introduction: body and soul! Contemporary art and healing. In: Body and Soul. Contemporary art and healing. De Cordova Museum, Lincoln, p 19

Laing R D 1965 The divided self. Penguin, Middlesex

Lather P 1991 Getting smart: feminist research and pedagogy within the postmodern. Routledge, New York

Lawlis F 1996 Transpersonal medicine. Shambala, Boston

Leininger M 1981 Caring: an essential need. Charles B Slack, Thorofare

Levin J 1993 Esoteric vs exoteric explanations for findings linking spirituality and health. Advances in Nursing Science 9(14):54–56

Lewenson S B 1996 Taking charge: nursing, suffrage and feminism in America, 1873–1920. National League for Nursing, New York, p ix

Lindburgh A M 1944 The steep ascent. Dell Books, New York

Lopez B 1989 Crossing open ground. Vintage Books, New York

Macrae J 1995 Nightingale's philosophy and its significance for modern nursing. Image: Journal of Nursing Scholarship 27(1):8–10

Malkin J 1992 Hospital interior architecture? Creating healing environments for special patient populations. Van Nostrand Reinhold, New York

Marcuse M 1977 The aesthetic dimension. Beacon Press, Boston

Margenau H 1987 The miracle of existence. Shambhala, New Science Library, Boston

Martin J R 1994 Changing the educational landscape: philosophy, women and curriculum. Routledge, London, p 38

McKivergin D, Daubenmire J 1994 The essence of therapeutic presence. Journal of Holistic Nursing 12(1):65–81

McNeill B (ed) Fall 1987 Editor's comments. Noetic Sciences Review 4:19

McNiff S 1992 Art as medicine. Shambala Publications, Boston, p 21

Mentgen J, Trapp, Bulbrook M J 1994 Healing touch. North Carolina Center for Healing Touch, Carrabarro

Merleau-Ponty, M 1962 Phenomenology of perception. Translated by Smith C, Routledge & Kegan Paul, London

Mitchell D P 1996 Postmodernism, health and illness. Journal of Advanced Nursing. 23:201–205

Mitchell G 1991 Nursing diagnosis: an ethical analysis. Image 23(2):99–103

Mitchell G, Santopinto M 1988 An alternative to nursing diagnosis. The Canadian Nurse 84(10):25–28

Moccia P 1994 Where do our loyalties lie? Nursing and Health Care 14(9): 472–474

Moore T 1992 Care of the soul. Harper Collins, New York

Muff J (ed) 1982 Socialization, sexism and stereotyping: women's issues in nursing. C V Mosby, St Louis

Muff J 1988 Of images and ideals: a look at socialization and sexism in nursing. In: Jones A H (ed) Images of nursing: perspectives from history, art and literature. University of Pennsylvania Press, Philadelphia, pp 197–220

Mumford L 1970 The myth of the machine. Harcourt Brace Jovanovich, New York, p 420

Murdock M 1990 The heroine's journey. Shambhala Publications, Boston

Murphy M 1992 The future of the body: explorations into the further evolution of human nature. J P Tarcher, Los Angeles

Muschamp X New York Times, 1995, p 38

Myss C 1996 Anatomy of the spirit. Harmony Books, New York

New King James Bible. 1611 1 Corinthians 6:19. Gideon International

Newman M 1992 Prevailing paradigms in nursing. Nursing Outlook 40(1):10–13, 32

Newman M 1994 Health as expanding consciousness. National League for Nursing, New York

Newman M, Sime M A, Corcoran-Perry S A 1991 The focus of the discipline of nursing. Advances in Nursing Science 14(1):1–6

Nightingale F 1859 (1992 commemorative edn) Notes on nursing. Introduction by B Barnum, commentaries by contemporary nursing leaders. J P Lippincott, Philadelphia

Nightingale F 1979 Cassandra: an essay. Feminist Press, Old Westbury

Noddings N 1989 Women and evil. University of California Press, Berkeley

Olness K, Mize W 1996 Intention and the awareness of the body. Advances in Nursing Science 12(3):23–26

O'Reagan B 1987 Healing, remission and miracle cures. Institute of Noetic Sciences special report. Noetic Sciences Institute, Sausalito

Overman 1986 The potentiation of healing: nursing's healing art. Unpublished manuscript, doctoral theory course. University of Colorado School of Nursing, Denver

Parses R 1981 Man-living-health: a theory of nursing. Wiley, New York

Parsons S 1917 'Addresses'—23rd Annual Conference, NLWE. Williams & Wilkins, Baltimore, p 56. In: Leweson S B 1996 Taking charge. Nursing, suffrage and feminism in America, 1873–1920. National League for Nursing, New York, Preface, p ix

Pehnt W 1991 Rudolf Steiner: Goetheanum, Dornach. Verlag Ernst & Sohn, Berlin, pp 56 and 71

Pelletier K R 1985 Toward a science of consciousness. Celestial Arts, Berkeley, p 55, 59, 66

Peter E, Gallop R 1994 The ethic of care: a comparison of nursing and medical students. Image: Journal of Nursing Scholarship 26(1):47–52

Playboy, November 1983 In: Jones A H (ed) 1988 Images of nursing: perspectives from history, art and literature. University of Pennsylvania Press, Philadelphia

Pribram K 1982 What the fuss is all about. In: Wilber K (ed) The holographic paradigm and other paradoxes. New Science Library, Boston

Proust M 1925 Remembrance of things past: the Guermanta way. Random House, New York

Quinn J 1996 The intention to heal: perspectives of a therapeutic touch practitioner and researcher. Advances in Nursing Science 12(3):26–29

Ray M 1994 Complex caring dynamics. A unifying model of nursing theory. Theoretical and Applied Chaos in Nursing 1(1):23–32

Reed P G 1991 Towards a nursing theory of self-transcendence. Advances in Nursing Science 13(4):64–77

Reed P G 1995 A treatise on nursing knowledge: development for the 21st century. Beyond postmodernism. Advances in Nursing Science 17(3):70–84

Remen R 1994 The recovery of the sacred: some thoughts on medical reform. ReVision 16(3):123–129

Reverby S 1987 A caring dilemma: womanhood and nursing in historical perspective. Nursing Research 36(1):5–10

Rogers M E 1970 A theoretical basis of nursing. F A Davis, Philadelphia

Rogers M E 1992 Prelude to 21st Century. In: Nightingale F 1992 commemorative edn Notes on nursing. J B Lippincott, Philadelphia

Rossman M 1996 Intentionality and healing. Advances 12(3):29–31

Rossner 1989 In: Harman W 1991 A reexamination of the metaphysical foundations of modern science. Institute of Noetic Sciences Review 4:22–25

Sacks O 1990 Seeing voices. Harper Perennial, New York

Sacks O 1995 An anthropologist on Mars: seven paradoxical tales. Alfred A Knopf, New York

Sarter B 1987 Evolutionary idealism:a philosophical foundation for holistic nursing theory. Advances in Nursing Science 9(2):1–9

Sartre J P 1963 Literature and existentialism. Citadel, New York

Sarup M 1988 Post-structuralism and postmodernism. Harvester Wheatsheaf, London

Schlitz M 1996a Intentionality and intuition and their implications: a challenge for science and medicine. The Journal of Mind-Body Health 12(2):58–66

Schlitz M 1996b Intentionality: a program of study. The Journal of Mind-Body Health 12(3):31–32

Shamansky S L, Yanni C R 1983 Opposition to nursing diagnosis: a minority opinion. Image 15:47–50

Shatchakra-Nirupanam 1931 A description of the six bodily centers of the unfolding serpent power. Translated by Avalon A. Ganesh Publications, Madras, India

Shepherd L J 1993 Lifting the veil: the feminine face of science. Shambhala Publications, Boston

Smith H 1982 Beyond the postmodern mind. Crossroads Publications, New York

Smith-Rosenberg C 1975 The female world of love and ritual. SIGNS: Journal of Women in Culture and Society August:1. [also in: Reverby S 1987 Nursing Research 36(1):7–10]

Sperry R 1987 Downward causation: the consciousness revolution in science. Noetic Sciences Review 4:18–21

Steinbeck J 1951 The log from the Sea of Cortez. Viking Press, New York

Steven S W 1953 Selected poems. Faber & Faber, London

Tarnas R 1993 The passion of the western mind: understanding the ideas that have shaped our worldview. Ballantine Books, New York

Taveira T 1990 Tomas Taveira: architectural works and design. Academy Editions, St Martin's Press, New York

Teilhard de Chardin P 1959 The phenomenon of man. Harper & Row, New York

Teilhard de Chardin P 1964 The future of man. Harper & Row, New York

Thomas L 1974 The lives of a cell. Bantam, New York

Thomas L 1984 Late night thoughts on listening to Mahler's ninth symphony. Bantam, New York

Thompson J D 1981 The passionate humanist: from Nightingale to the new nurse. In: Florence Nightingale: saint, reformer or rebel? Robert E Krieger, Malabar, pp 220–230

Toulmin S 1990 Cosmopolis. The hidden agenda of modernity. The Free Press, Macmillan, New York

Van de Vanter L, Fuey J A (eds) 1991 Vision of war, dreams of peace. Warner Books, New York, p 201

Vaughn F 1986 The inward arc. Shambhala, New Science Library, Boston

Walker M 1937, 1942 (rev edn 1975) For my people. In: Norton Anthology of Poetry. W W Norton, New York, p 1168

Watkins A D 1995 Perception, emotions and immunity: an integrated homeostatic network. Quarterly Journal of Medicine 88:283–294

Watkins A D 1996 Intention and the electromagnetic activity of the heart. The Journal of Mind-Body Health 12(3):35–36

Watson J 1979 Nursing: the philosophy and science of caring. Little Brown, Boston. Reprinted 1985 Colorado Associated Press, Boulder

Watson J 1987 Nursing on the caring edge: metaphorical vignettes. Advances in Nursing Science 10(1):10–18

Watson J 1988a New dimensions of human caring theory. Nursing Science Quarterly 1(4):175–181

Watson J 1988b Nursing: human science and human care. National League for Nursing, New York

Watson J 1989 The moral failure of the patriarchy. Nursing Outlook 28(2):62–66

Watson J 1992a University of Colorado Center for Human Caring brochure. Denver

Watson J 1992b Guidelines for caring then and now. In: Nightingale F 1992 commemorative edn Notes on nursing. Introduction by Barnum B, commentaries by contemporary nursing leaders, J B Lippincott, Philadelphia

Watson J 1995 Postmodernism and knowledge development in nursing. Nursing Science Quarterly 8(2):60–64

Weber R 1982 Field consciousness and field ethics. In: Wilber K (ed) 1982 The holographic paradigm and other paradoxes. New Science Library, Boston

Weber R 1986 Dialogues with scientists and sages: the search for unity. Routledge and Kegan Paul, London

Whitehead A N 1953 Science and the modern world. Cambridge University Press

Wilber K 1981 No boundary. Shambhala Publications, Boston

Wilber K (ed) 1982 The holographic paradigm and other paradoxes. New Science Library, Boston

Wolfe T 1987 From Bauhaus to our house. Penguin, London

Woolf V 1938 Three guineas. Harcourt Brace Jovanovich, San Diego

Woolf V 1976 Moments of being. Harcourt Brace Jovanovich, New York

Young S 1994 Purpose and method of Vipassana meditation. The Humanistic Psychologist 22:53–61

Zeiger A 1960 Afterword to Jane Eyre, 3rd edn. New American Library of World Literature, New York, p 459

Zukav G 1990 The seat of the soul. Fireside: Simon and Schuster, New York

Glossary of definitions

Archetypal The adjective for archetype, referring to the basic ancestor form and image of humanity laid in our collective human unconscious, from our collective ancestors. (See Archetype.)

Archetype An enduring unconscious idea, image, original form or pattern in the human consciousness that is present and persists across time and across humanity; the origin of meaning in humanity is from Jungian psychology, which posits that basic forms (archetypal images) are inherited from our ancestors and the human race; these forms and intrinsic meanings associated with the human condition transcend age, race, culture and nation. Such a basic concept emerges individually and collectively in society and humanity; archetype transcends the postmodern trend that critiques and rejects universals. Archetype and archetypal hold paradoxical meanings for the postmodern era; they are both timeless and yet subject to critique and challenge. The archetype underpins the basic search for wholeness, beauty and harmony sought within the postmodern critique.

Archetypes are one form of inner knowing and a timeless yet time-experienced truth, which are in the world but also stand beyond it. An archetype is a timeless path to human and natural existence, perhaps to existence in the universe. It is a basic energy and form of being. Archetype constitutes the veiled essence of things (Tarnas 1993, p. 6). In a fundamental form, what we perceive in the world is better understood as a concrete expression of a more fundamental idea, an archetype, which gives special structure, condition and deeper meaning to the thing itself.

Despite the reality of archetypal levels of existence and being, the ordinary person is not directly aware of an archetype or archetypal meanings that inform his or her day-to-day life. In art and poetry for example, the artist unveils the authentic reality behind the appearance; one participates in the absolute 'form of beauty' (Tarnas 1993, p. 8). The archetype is apparent not so much to the limited physical senses, though these can suggest and lead the way, but to the more penetrating eye of the soul, the illuminated intellect. Archetypes thus reveal themselves more to the inner perception than to the outer. There is a sense of the dynamic universal: transcending but also embodying the essence contained within the image/ metaphor itself. However, to engage in archetypal insights and wisdom, one needs to 'awaken' to a more profound level of reality, and to a deeper mindfulness of intuition, sacredness, unconsciousness and mindfulness of being.

The caring and deep feminine energy of nursing as metaphor connects at the deep archetypal level within a professional health context, but also for humanity. Nursing/caring can be considered a feminine archetype of nurturance, sustenance, connectedness, loving, protection, birthing and flowing of natural life processes; healing the primordial wound of humankind, nature and life-giving processes. While perfect caring may not exist, nursing and nurse stand as an archetypal, metaphorical form of feminine, life-giving, caring–healing processes. It is both time-bound and timeless. It is far from being unreal, an abstraction or imaginary metaphor for the concrete world of medical care practices. It is considered here (as well as in Tarnas' work) to be the very basis of reality. It is the sacred feminine archetype, contained in nursing's caring–healing model, which determines its order and renders it knowable and capable of manifestation at the professional, institutional and cultural level.

Cosmological and cosmological shift Refers to changing views of what it means to be human in the universe; the cosmos; the shift refers to changing human mindset still adhering to stable, unchanging laws of the universe to notions of evolving consciousness in relation to an expanding universe; notions of relativity of time, space, causality and physicality emerge; cosmological shift also implies a reconsideration of what it means to be human in a changing universe. Cosmological shift in thinking implies the concept of evolving human consciousness, and evolving human as an integral part of the universe, not standing outside of it seeking to control and be dominant, but to understand and be in harmony with the whole cosmos.

Covolution Where all living things self-organize and evolve through mutual dependency—a symbiotic dance, in which species co-evolve (Briggs & Peat 1990, p 160).

Deconstructed Taking apart, dismantling; used in postmodern literature to imply dismantling of ideas, mindsets, relationships, hierarchies, power–gender imbalances, critiquing of texts, meanings and social norms and established 'modern' worldview. [Author note: some postmodern critiques engage in deconstruction of meaning, without necessarily seeking a constructive reconstruction of thinking, leaving only the dismantled version of critique.] In postmodern literature, deconstruct refers to a close reading of a text, to critique not only what is said but also what is not said: what resides in the margins of the text and is implied in the context of the whole. Deconstruction of text and meaning can be both liberating and insightful, but it can also create an unraveling of social and scientific reality, resulting in moral anarchy (Watson 1995).

Empirical Refers to knowledge and ways of knowing and determining values about what is known and what is reliable to know—that is, empirical data are derived from sense data, observation and experiments alone; data which are provable and verifiable in the concrete physical–material world. Empirical data do not accommodate theory nor philosophy nor metaphysical concepts, unless they are verifiable and confirmed by experiment and observation.

Epistemologies   That which pertains to nature of knowledge, ways of knowing and how one knows what one knows; technically (Webster's encyclopedic unabridged dictionary of the English language 1989. Gramercy Book, New Jersey, p 480) 'a branch of philosophy that investigates the origin, nature, methods and limits of human knowledge'.

Epistemic   Refers to knowledge and conditions for obtaining knowledge and ways of knowing.

Intersubjective   The coming together of two or more persons interacting through their unique subjective human realities; two persons' consciousness co-mingling to create new meaning; a new entity of meaning, greater than, and different from, two separate objective persons communicating or relating. The uniting of two or more persons' subjective realities to create a new perspective; that which emerges out of the shared relationship and inner unique life world of their subjective perceptions and experiences.

Metaphysical   Beyond the physical; that which pertains to one's view of reality which embraces both matter and spirit and is concerned with abstract thought, existence and philosophical; technically 'a branch of philosophy that includes ontology, cosmology, and epistemology and its abstract branches' (Webster's encyclopedic unabridged dictionary of the English language 1989. Gramercy Book, New Jersey, p 901).

Modern   The dominant mindset of the 20th century; belief systems and values with the following themes: science, objectivity, rationality, physical–material world, linear cause and effect, industrial product-line thinking, technology, machines, empirical knowledge, belief in universal principles and stable laws; also within context of history it refers to contemporary times, the present age; modern Western thinking has come to convey positivist reasoning with neutrality of human values (Watson 1995). This era is represented by dominant metaphors of machine-technology science and physical reality as supreme reality.

Ontological and ontological shift Refers to the meaning of 'being'; raising questions about what it means to be human, to be healed, to be cured, to be caring and cared for; a basic change of consciousness about 'being' which moves from 'being human', implying separate, independent individuals, disconnected from self–other–environment–nature–universe, to reconsidering the meaning of 'being human' in relation with and seeking harmony with all else in the universe.

Postmodern No one meaning is possible; postmodern refers to and is used, in this text, as: (1) a periodizing concept capturing this moment in human history which goes beyond—'past' this modern era and opens to a new period in human history; (2) the beginning and end of modernity (Watson 1995); (3) the emergent, dynamic, changing perspective and intellectual movement that critiques and actually rejects the dominant mindset of the 'modern' era; (4) the emerging postmodern mindset suggests there is no one Truth, but multiple truths; no one universally known reality that is defined by physical–material world; rather, there are multiple, constructed realities, there is attention to valuing multiple meanings; acknowledgment of both physical and non-physical reality and phenomena; the postmodern suggests non-linearity of thinking and acting, introduces relativity of time and space; is open to ideas that include context, critiques, challenges, multiple interpretations, stories, narratives, text and search for meaning and wholeness. Emerging metaphors of postmodern: art, artistry, creativity, harmony, beauty, spirit-metaphysical, holographic.

Praxis   Refers to informed practice; integrative practice informed by one's values, intentionality, consciousness, one's ethic and full self. Caring–healing praxis integrates doing, knowing and being into transformative caring, healing and health care within a given moment.

Quantum   A term from physics and quantum mechanics, now more commonly used in lay language, referring to a speed and velocity associated with the speed of light; a highly rapid amount and quantity of energy movement that exceeds and transcends common logic. As in quantum jump, or quantum leap, implying high speed that is beyond what one might imagine or comprehend.

Reconstructed   Putting back together in new patterns and order of relationships resulting in new meaning and evolved, expanded mindsets, and new values. The terminology is found in postmodern literature along with deconstructed. This text seeks to uncover and deconstruct the difficulties of the modern medical mindset, while moving beyond the deconstruction towards a reconstruction of positive ideas and hopeful thinking, resulting in transformation. The other side of deconstruction, a search for meaning that brings an emergence of wholeness, beauty, and connectedness and higher evolution (Watson 1995).

Transpersonal   Conveys a human-to-human connection (usually in a caring moment), in which both persons are influenced through the relationship and the being together in a given moment; transpersonal conveys a human connection, beyond personal body-physical ego, and has a spiritual dimension; it implies a focus on the uniqueness of self and other coming together, moving from the fully embodied physical ego-self to deeper, more spiritual, transcendent even cosmic connections that tap into healing; transpersonal includes the unique individuality of each human, while extending beyond the ego-self, radiating and transcending to deeper connections all humans share with their deeper selves, other, environment, nature and the universe. (See Watson's theory of transpersonal caring 1996 In: Walker P H, Neuman B (eds) 1996 Blueprint for use of nursing models. National League for Nursing, New York, pp 141–184.)

Yang   Refers to masculine energy and its associated principles. Literally 'the sunny side of the mountain'; one of the two fundamental polar [archetypal] forces that organize the universe. Yang manifests itself as form, light, noise, warmth, activity; (from Beinfield H, Korngold E 1992 Between heaven and earth. Ballantine, New York, p 411.) (author's parenthesis).

Yin   Refers to feminine energy and its associated principles. Literally 'the shady side of the mountain'; one of the two fundamental polar [archetypal] forces that organize the universe. Yin manifests as substance, darkness, quietness, coldness; (from Beinfield H, Korngold E 1992 Between heaven and earth. Ballantine, New York, p 412.) (author's parenthesis).

Index

Page numbers in **bold** indicate figures and tables. Page numbers in *italic* indicate illustrations in the color section.

Aboriginal dreamtime 23
Acorn and oak tree, metaphor 123, 153
Active imagery 211
Actual caring occasion 116–117
Acupressure 216
Advanced practice
  boundary concerns 43
  changing role 39–40
AIDS/HIV, nurse-managed center for 190–191
Air quality, healing environment 252
The Alchemist 31
Alternative medicine *see* Complementary medicine
Altruism and autonomy 35
Ambiguity, quantum 122
American Holistic Nursing Association xxiv
American hospitals, hierarchical system 78
American Nurses' Association (ANA)
  Definition and Social Policy Statement 40, 41
  revised definition of nursing 44
An Anthropologist on Mars, Sacks 143–144
Ancient wisdom 60–73
Anthroposophic architecture 250, **251**
Anthroposophy, Steiner 250
Applied kinesiology **223**
Archetype and archetypal, definitions 285–286
Archetypes
  see also The sacred feminine
  archetypal dimension, nursing 10
    see also Nursing: as archetype and metaphor
  and collective unconsciousness, Jung 151–152
Architecture
  and art 270
  caring-healing 243–259
  environment, effects of 243
  healing art in 196–197, 198–199
  modern **244**
  premodern **244**

rethinking urban issues 52–53
  symbolic and sacred archetypal 254–255
Aromatherapy 212, 214, 249
Art
  and architecture 270
  and beauty 193–200
  and cancer 197–198
  in healing, categories 195–197
  and healing, new relationship between 195
  and science, reintegration 195
  therapeutic-healing value 197–198, 199
Auditory modalities, intentional conscious use 206–209
  postmodern/transpersonal caring arts 207–209
  premodern Nightingale 206–207
Australia, ontological shift, nursing education and practice 188
Authoritarianism, nursing education 36–37
Autopsy, introducing medical students to 132–133
Awareness, primordial energy, *Sacred Mirrors* 11

Backstage/centerstage metaphor, Herbert 107–108
Bauhaus school of architecture 245, 247
Beauty and art 193–200
  in healing practices 194–195
Bed as metaphor 238
Bedmaking, Zen of 237–240
Belief systems, importance 119
Benor, subtle biological energy 124
The blade, power metaphor 58
Blake, concept of body 131
Boat, Steinbeck's 4
The body
  connecting with, exercise 172–175
  and consciousness 133–134
  as living energy field 160
  modern sense of 134
  normative medical approach 135–136
  and personhood, extraordinary dimensions 141–142
  postmodern/transpersonal 124–125, 131–157, **135**, **146–147**

The body *(cont'd)*
  as sacred mirror 159–169
  as subject 138–139
  as temple 229–230
Body therapy/touch therapy 216
  additional therapies **223–224**
Body-ego self and transpersonal self,
    comparison **156**
Body-physical model of human 132
Bodywork fields 222
Bohm
  creative play of the universe 123
  moment of consciousness 117
  moments of time 105
  quantum notion of connectedness
      108–109
  unbroken wholeness 95, 98
Brazil, ontologocal shift, nursing education
    and practice 189
Breast cancer and art 197–198
Bronte, *Jane Eyre* 138–140, 141–142
Buddha, teachings of 238
Byrd, prayer and coronary patients,
    study 120

Campbell
  oneness of all 153
  sacred and soul, loss of 86
  war, greatest works of 69
Canada, ontologically based nursing practices
    and scholarship 185–186
Cancer and art 197–198
Candlelight ritual 272, 273–276
Care in modern nursing 181
Caring
  acts, postmodern/transpersonal framework
      239–240
  basis and value of 38
  consciousness 179, 226, 230
    and healing consciousness 148–151
    holographic 109, 120
    intentional use of 224–227
    premodern Nightingale 224–225
  cosmology 3
  ethic 64, 65, 67
  field and caring moment **114**, 118
  literature 100
  model, transpersonal 154–157
  moment 11, 113, 116–118, 149
    and caring field **114**, 118
    holographic 109–114
    transpersonal 114, 115–118
  as moral ideal 68, 265
  in nursing 10, 11, 128
  as ontology 65, 179, 191
  practices, from carative factors 264
  touch 216

Caring-healing 268
  architecture 243–259
  art within perspective of 195
  arts, professional ontological competencies
      as 201–233
  consciousness 111, 179
  cosmology 94–95
  dimensions of nursing xxi
  energy of nursing 6
  Era III/Paradigm III, 102–104
  modalities 204–205, 206–227
  model xxv, xxv-xxvi, 88–89, 264–265
  moment *see* Caring: moment
  paradigm 95, **96**, 265
  postmodern reconstruction 20
  professional models 85
  relational spiritual aspect 180
  transformative model 102
  transpersonal xxv, 105–130
Center for Human Caring, Colorado
    see University of Colorado Center
    for Human Caring
Centering 216
  exercise 171–172
Chakra system 161–162
  color therapy 161–162, 249
  Myss 163–164
    energy and anatomy **165–166**, **167**
  Sacred Mirrors, Grey 9–*10*
The Chalice and the Blade, Eisler 61
The chalice, metaphor 58
Changing roles, external pressures 39–40
Chardin, Teilhard de 3, 5, 95, 105, 128,
    155, 171
Charity *1*
Chinese proverb 269
Chiropractic **223**
A Chorus of Stones: the Private Life of War,
    Griffin 62, 63
Collective unconsciousness xx-xxi, 151–152
Color
  chakras 161–162, 249
  use, healing environment 253
Communication, healing environment 252
Competition and jealousy in nursing 43–44
Complementary medicine 100–101
  aromatherapy 212, 214, 249
Complexity science 125–126, 128
Concrescence 114, 117
Connectedness
  with human spirit 117
  quantum theory 108–109
Connecting with the body exercise 172–175
Conscious intentionality 146–147
Consciousness
  as energy 179
  energy and light, relationship 111–113, 121,
      147, 148, 256

evolving 128, 143, 146, 230
higher states 123
holographic theory 109
and intentionality 121–123
  in mind-body research 123–128
modalities 221
moment of 117
non-local 120, 142
ontological shift 56
paradigm, reconsidering nursing
    therapeutics within 228–229
reconsidering caring and healing
    consciousness 148–151
shared 118
universal, and the sacred unconscious
    151–153
Cooperation, sacred feminine archetype
    232
Cosmic-earth process, humans as expression
    of 80
Cosmological and cosmological shift,
    definitions 286–287
Cosmology 11
  see also The sacred feminine
  caring 3
  caring-healing 94–95
  emerging, postmodern discourse 126
  metaphors reflecting prevailing 59–60
  of oneness of consciousness 97–98
  postmodern era 78
  sacred archetype 230
  Western cultural 15
Costs, low nursing salaries to contain 45
Covolution 54, 55, 287
Crete, ancient culture 60
Cultural value difference, men/women,
    medicine/nursing 78
Cyberspace and virtual space 142–143

Davidson, healing space and the environment
    248
Death experience and music 208
Deconstrucing/reconstructing process 97
Deconstruction 19–21
  definition 19, 287
  the modern 95
  modern metaphors 57–73
  modern nursing 33–47
Definitions of nursing, ANA 40, 41, 44
The Denver Nursing Project in Human Caring
    190–191
Derrida, deconstruction 19
Diagnosis and treatment as power words
    40–41
Diagnostic process
  potential harm 41–42
  related to pathophysiological event 42

Dominator model 15, 57–58, 61, 69
  breakdown of system 59
Donoghue, text and margin 17
Dossey
  *Healing Words, the Power of Prayer
    and the Practice of Medicine* 120
  non-local consciousness 120, 142
Dreaming 23–27

Eastern traditions, consciousness and
    energy 106
  see also Chakra system; Yang; Yin;
    Yin-Yang system
Educational
  entry points and intraprofessional
    jealousy 44
  reform 69
Ego self to transpersonal self 155–157
Eisler, *The Chalice and the Blade* 61
The emerging human 146–147
Emerson, beauty 193
Empirical, definition 287–288
Energy
  consciousness and caring 105–109, 229
  meridian 216
  and thought processes 106
Energy-based therapeutics 217
Environmental
  effects, health and healing 202–203, 243,
    250, 253
  essentials 249
  health 213
Epistemic and epistemologies, definitions 288
Epochal
  evolution 81–82
  shift, Western mind 56
Eras, medical science and treatment models
    98
  Era I 98–99
  Era II 98, 99–100
  Era III 98, 101, 104, 110, 111, 113, 125,
    126, 129, 151, 191–192, 271
Evolution
  beyond five-sensory human 146
  direction of 54, 59, 128, 143, 154
  epochal 81–82
  evolving
    consciousness 128, 143, 146, 230
    medical health-care approaches **178**
    worldview **2**
Evolutionary process, Nightingale and
    Era III/Paradigm III thinking 203
Exercises, experiencing transpersonal body
    171–175
Expert knowledge 18
The extrasensory human 141–146
Extrasensory perceptual abilities 144–145

Families, accommodation in healing environments 253
Feelings, sacred feminine archetype 231
Feldenkrais 223
Female symbol, Venus's mirror 49, 50
The feminine
  see also The sacred feminine
  repression of 51, 85–86
  revaluing principle 84
  Yin 77
Feminine creativity, ancient cultures 60–61
Feminine perspective 65
  emergence, public consciousness 52
  growing interest in 53–54
  Western medicine, lack of 14–16
Field of consciousness 229
Fight ethic, modern medicine 57, 58
Foot reflexology 216
Fox, 12th century mystic prophets 61–62
The Future of the Body, Murphy 138–139, 141

Gablik
  modern and postmodern art 194
  traditions, modern art world 193
Gadamer, The Relevance of the Beautiful 193–194
Gahrton, male-dominated society 63
Glossary of definitions 285–291
Goodman, revisionist medicine 67–68
Greene
  the arts 194
  invisible world 24–25, 26
  'wide awakeness' 126–127
Grey, Alex
  mystical experience, body as energy 11, 168–169
  Sacred Mirrors 7, 8, 9, 10, 11, 159–167, 168, 196
Griffin
  A Chorus of Stones: the Private Life of War 62, 63
  public and private events 37
  the soul 82
Griffiths, peace to end all wars 63
Gustatory modalities, intentional conscious use of 218–220
  postmodern/transpersonal caring arts 219–220
  premodern Nightingale 218–219

Handwashing, Zen of 239
Harman, higher states of consciousness 123
Healing
  arts, categories 195–197
  arts and the nurse/healing practitioner 193–200

environment 248–249, 250
  Malkin, guide to developing 250, 252–253
  nature of 30–31
  practices, beauty and art in 194–195
  touch 217–218
'Healing temple' architecture 251
Healing Words, the Power of Prayer and the Practice of Medicine, Dossey 120
Health care reforms, late 20th century 101–102
Heidegger, path towards the light 24
Herbert
  backstage/centerstage metaphor 107–108
  quantum ambiguity 122
Hermeneutic study, nursing textbooks, Hiraki 70–72
Hierarchical
  nature, institutional culture 45, 78
  structure, Western cultural cosmology 15
  system 69
  versus complementary system 75–76
Higher education, 1960s 72
Higher states of consciousness 123
Hildegard of Bingen 12, 169–170
Hiraki, hermeneutic study, introductory nursing textbooks 70–72
Historical periods of major transitions 9
Holism, Pribram 108
Holographic metaphorical model 107, 109
  caring moment 109–114
  image, eagle 5
  model of caring consciousness 120
  thinking, basic principles 110
Hospitals
  for the 21st century 254, 255, 256, 257, 258
  and public institutions, modern architecture 248
Human autopsy experience, introducing medical students to 132–133
Human consciousness see Consciousness
Human-nature-universe relationships 19
Human/environment oneness xxii

Identity and boundaries 37–46
  questions of 38, 39
Inner, architecture 52–53
Inner light, choosing to follow 28–29
Institutional
  culture 45
  nursing xx, xxi
Integrative-interactive paradigm see Paradigms: nursing: paradigm II
Intention 216
  and consciousness, Zukav 148

Intentionality 119–121
  actions and effects 147
  and consciousness 121–123
  and evolution 146
  mind-body research 123–128
  toward sacred healing 230
Internal grids of reference *see* Lens
Intersection between
  masculine and feminine principles
    83–84
  planes of existence 78, 79
  world and time 80–87
Intersubjective, definition 288
Intuiting, developing, sacred feminine
    archetype 232
Involuntary memories, smell 213

Jackson, metaphors of falling and
    disequilibrium 136–137
James, William, postmodern transpersonal
    orientation towards body 135
Janck, postmodern architecture 243, 245
Jane Eyre, Bronte 138–140, 141–142
Jin Shin Jyutsu 223
Journal entry, Venus's mirror 62–63
Jung, archetypes and collective unconscious
    151–152

Kadinsky, art and the spiritual 195
Kaiser, hospitals for the 21st century 254, 255,
    256, 257, 258
Kech, epochal evolution 81–82
Keller, Helen, extrasensory perceptual abilities
    144–145
Kinesthetic modalities, intentional conscious
    use 221–224
  postmodern/transpersonal caring arts
    222–224
  premodern Nightingale 221–222
Knowledge base needed by nurses, Nightingale
    201–202
Knowledge and science, Western tradition 69
Kofutu touch healing 223
Krysl, *Poem for the left and right hand* 30
Kundalini 162
Kung
  science and spirit 108
  values 104

Language
  see also Metaphors
  diagnostic process and power 42
  hermeneutic study, nursing textbooks
    70–71
  jargon, isolation of nursing 36

masculine gender word 51
  and power, adoption of terminology
    40–41, 44
  of war 12
  see also Fight ethic, modern medicine
Lather, redefinition of nursing 47
The left and right hand 29–31
Lens 85
  changing the 87–88
Levin, spirituality and health outcomes 119
Light
  healing environment 252
  as metaphor 271–272
  and ritual, metaphors and symbols for
    nursing 269
Lindburgh
  peace and war 60
  planes of existence 78
Lomi 223
Loving and caring, sacred feminine archetype
    232

Mackintosh, Charles Rennie 245
McKivergin and Daubenmire, concept of
    presence 225–226
McNiff
  art 195, 199
  shamanic cultures 197
Male
  dominated society, Gahrton 63
  perspective, Western intellectual tradition
    50–51
Malkin, healing environments 248–249, 250,
    252–253
Marcuse, world of inner life 25
Margenau, evolving humanity 154
MariEL 223
Martin, ontological basement 34
Masculine archetype 29–30
  institutional reflection of 73
  modern medicine 14
  Western intellectual tradition 50–51
  Yang 77
Masculine and feminine
  perspectives, reconciliation 54–55
  principles, intersection 83–84
  symbols 49, **50**
Matter and energy, complementarity 106
Media sterotypes of nursing 34–35
Medical cure model 132
  deconstruction 20
Medical science 8
  cosmology 15
  hierarchical structure, power/knowledge 18
Medical-health care approaches, evolving
    178
Medicalization, caring process 42

Medicine
  see also Eras, medical science and treatment
      models; Paradigms: nursing
  masculine archetype of 14
  as masculine energy 76
  and nursing, gap between 66–67
Meditation
  or prayer 229
  for transpersonal/postmodern body and self
      167–170
Mental-cognitive modalities, intentional use
      220–221
  postmodern/transpersonal caring arts 221
  premodern Nightingale 220–221
Metaphor and metamorphosis, Steven 270
Metaphors 12–13
  acorn and oak tree 123, 153
  backstage/centerstage 107–108
  bed as 238
  being 'off-balance' 136–137
  the blade, power metaphor 58
  Boat, Steinbeck 4
  the chalice, receptivity and harmonization
      58
  consciousness and energy seen as 106
  deconstructing modern 57–73
  holographic model see Holographic
      metaphorical model
  of human movement 137
  light 271–272
    and ritual 269
  nursing as 49, 88
  power 58
  reflecting prevailing cosmology 59–60
  sea 5
  of war 12
Metaphysical
  definition 288
  mirrors for physical conditions 256
Millenium as coming of age 81
Mind, need for knowledge of 262–263
Mind-body research, transpersonal
      consciousness and intentionality
      123–128
Mindbodyspirit unity xxii, xxvi, 97–98
  values-based approach to nursing 263–264
Mindful presence 179
Moccia
  nurses and higher education 72
  nursings' loyalties 72–73
  questions posed for nursing 46
Models for nursing
  false boundaries 39
  postmodern and beyond 102–104
Modern
  architecture 243, 244, 245, 247
    hospitals and public institutions 248
  definition 288–289

medicine, the masculine archetype 29–30
  nursing, deconstructing 33–47
  to postmodern transition 4, 88–89
Modern/postmodern juncture 8–9
Moments of possibilities 122
  see also Caring: moments
Moral
  see also Values
  courage 68
  ideal, caring as 265
Muff
  adoption of roles in nursing 43–44
  authoritarianism, nursing education 37
  disagreement and progress in nursing 36
  identity and boundaries 38
  rivalry for power 44
  stereotypes of nurses 34–35
Multiplicity, sacred feminine archetype 232
Mumford
  modern/postmodern juncture 9
  transformation and self 104
Murdock, nursing, connecting with the sacred
      feminine 27, 28–29
Murphy
  The Future of the Body 138–139, 141–142
  transformative capacity 144
Music and sound in healing 206
Myss, Chakra system 163–164
  energy and anatomy 164–166
Mystic prophets, 12th century 61–62
Myth and ritual 270

National Institutes of Health Office of
      Complementary-Alternative Medicine
      (NIH-OCAM) 100–101
Negative emotions 111, 147
  mind-body research 124
Nervous system, Sacred Mirrors, Grey 8
Neuromuscular release 223
New Zealand, ontological shift, nursing
      education and practice 188
Newman
  consciousness 118
  holographic model 107
  nurse-client relationship 204
  paradigm of unitary consciousness 125
  sharing of consciousness, professional
      practice 178
Nightingale 6
  bedmaking 237
  body as temple 229–230
  caring-healing modalities
    auditory 206–207
    caring consciousness 224–225
    gustatory 218–219
    kinesthetic 221–222
    mental-cognitive 220–221

olfactory 212
  tactile 214–215
  visual 209–210
caring-healing model 264–265
environment and healing 202–203, 250, 253
knowledge base needed by nurses 201–202
model or metaparadigm 230–231
Notes on Nursing 201, 250, 253, 258, 265
nurse's role 258
postmodern messages 267–268
and postmodern nursing 261–268
  health knowledge and wisdom 262
  human mind, need for knowledge of 262–263
premodern modalities and postmodern transpersonal caring-healing 205
reconsideration of 201–233
spiritual, non-physical realm 139
values-based approach 263
war 62
women's place in society 66
'Nightingalism' 43
Nodding, gap between medicine and nursing 66–67
Noise
  healing environment 252
  Nightingale 206
  reduction 249
Non-local consciousness, Dossey 120, 142
Non-physical self 149–150
Norway, ontological shift, nursing education and practice 187
Notes on Nursing, Nightingale 201, 250, 253, 258, 265
Nurse-client relationship 178, 204
  as shared consciousness 118
Nurses, as ontological architects 257–259
Nursing
  as archetype and metaphor 11, 14–15, 50, 51, 88
  authoritarianism in 36–37
  caring in 89
  caring-healing dimensions xxi
  definition, ANA 40–41, 44
  diagnosis, ethics of 41–42
  education 36, 37
  expanding or changing role 45–46
  as feminine energy 76
  images of 33–37
    as sterotype 33–34
  model, reconstructed 88–89, 102–104
  modern, deconstructing 33–47
  new paradigm 95, **96**
  as ontological artistry 231
  paradigm III models for research and scholarship 233
  paradigm case for women and healing 15

paradigm choices 233
philosophies and theories, dissonance in 38
in postmodern ontological shift 87
postmodern/transpersonal awareness and healing environments 255
practices, ontologically based 181–192
reconstructing 75–89
redefining 10, 47, 51, 52, 75–80, 88–89, 94–95
research within human science paradigm 100
science, 1980s 101
skills, Zen of 239–240
technical view of 71
textbooks, Hiraki's hermenueutic study 70–72
within traditional medical science xxii, xxiv
Nursing qua nursing paradigm xxi-xxii, 46–47, 52, 54–55, 129–130
see also Transpersonal: caring-healing: model
Nursing's
  contributions worldwide 44–45
  loyalties, Moccia 72–73
Nurturing, sacred feminine archetype 232

Olfactory modalities, intentional conscious use of 212–214
see also Smell
postmodern/transpersonal caring arts 212–214
premodern Nightingale 212
Olfactory receptor cell 213–214
Ontological
  architects, nurses as 257–259
  competencies
    of being 230
    for transpersonal practice 177–200
  definition 289
  design framework, architecture and healing environments 255
  insecurity 36
  shift 56, 94–95, 289
    ego self to transpersonal self 155–157
    evolving human potential 21
    international examples 187–189
    in postmodern world 87
    transpersonal perspective 149
    Zen awareness 240
Ontologically based nursing practices 181–192
  international/national nursing examples 182–186
Ontology
  caring as 179
  of relation 97

Paradigm shift, emergent 192
Paradigms
  modern medical *see* Eras, medical science
    and treatment models
  nursing
    paradigm I 98–99
    paradigm II 98, 99–100
    paradigm III 98, 101, 104, 110, 111, 113,
      125, 126, 129, 151, 191–192, 271
    possibilities, eras and evolutions 98–102
    postmodern and beyond 125
Particle and wave phenomena 107
Partnership model 61
  in health care 59
The Passion of the Western Mind, Tarnas
    69–70
Peace and caring, journal entry 63
Peace, sacred feminine archetype 232
Pelletier, quantum theory 106
Perspective, internal grids of refernce *see* Lens
Pew-Fetzer Task Group of Psychosocial
    Education, approach to autopsy study
    132–133
Physical presence 225–226
Planes of existence, intersection between
    78, 79
Playboy magazine 34
Poem for the left and right hand, Krysl 30
Polarity **223**
Portugal, ontologically based nursing practice
    and scholarship 182
Positive emotions 112, 147
Postmodern
  architecture 243, 245, **246**, 257
  challenge for nursing 46–47
  changes in medicine and nursing 55–56
  deconstruction, conventional medical model
    101–102
  deconstruction/reconstruction 19–22
  definition 289
  messages, Nightingale 267–268
  nursing
    meaning xxii-xxiii
    model of 86–87, 93–104
    task of 24
  reconstruction, beyond nursing model
    102–104
Postmodern/transpersonal
  architecture 254
  awareness in nursing 255
  body 6, 124–125, 131–157
    emerging explanatory view 146–147
    exercises for experiencing 171–175
  caring arts
    caring consciousness 225–227
    discussion 227–233
    gustatory modalities 219–220
    kinesthetic modalities 222–224

    mental-cognitive modalities 221
    olfactory modality 212–214
    tactile modality 215–218
    visual modality 210–212
  framework, nursing skills within 239–240
  health professionals and education 256
  nursing 269
Power
  the blade, metaphor 58
  and language 42, 44
    diagnosis and treatment, power words
      40–41
  medicine and nursing, inequites between 43
  power/knowledge nexus, medical science 18
  rivalry for 44
Praxis, definition 290
Prayer, influence on health 120, 229
Prehistory 60–73
Premodern architecture **244**
Presence, concept of 225–226
Pribram
  construction of hard reality 110
  holism 108
Privacy, healing environment 252
Procedural touch 216
Professional
  capabilities, alternative medicine
    177–178
  models of caring-healing 85
  ontological competencies as advanced
    caring-healing arts 201–233
  socialization 36, 37
'Psychic energy system', Grey 9, 161
Psychological presence 226
Psychoneuroimmunology (PNI) 100, 249
Public
  consciousness, emergence of feminine
    perspective 52
  health and human caring 266–267
  use of transpersonal caring-healing
    modalities 227–228

Quantum
  ambiguity 122
  caring field 109–114
  definition 290
  reality 127
  theory 106–109, 125–126
    connectedness 108–109
    reality 121

Rational approach to life 247
Ray, caring movement in nursing 128
Reality
  construction of 'hard' 110
  quantum 121, 127

Receptivity, sacred feminine archetype 232
Reconstructed, definition 290
Reconstruction 22
  nursing 75–89, 95, 97–98
Redefinition of nursing 10, 47, 51, 52, 75–80,
    88–89, 94–95
Reforms, health care systems 266–267
Reiki **224**
Relatedness, sacred feminine archetype 232
The Relevance of the Beautiful, Gadamer
    193–194
Relighting the lamp 269–276
Remen
  lack of feminine viewpoint 16
  the Yin 28
Reverby
  altruism and autonomy 35
  basis of caring 47
  metaphor of nursing 49
  nursing education 37
  power inequites, medicine and nursing 43
Revisionist medicine, Goodman 67–68
Ritual 269, 270, 276
  candlelight 272, 273–276
  recreating meaningful 258–259, 273–275
  and value system 270–271
Rogers
  Nightingale and postmodern caring-healing
      modalities 202
  technology, over-emphasis 201
  the unitary person 164
Role, change, response to external pressures
    39–40
Rolfing **224**

Sacks, *An Anthropologist on Mars.*
    Seven Paradoxical Tales 143–144
The sacred
  need for 83
  unconscious and universal consciousness
      151–153
Sacred archetype cosmology 230
The sacred feminine 6
  see also The feminine
  archetype 231–232
  cosmology 268
  healing 30–31
  nursing as archetype 11, 13, 22, 255
  in search of 23–31
  transpersonal caring-healing work 128
Sacred Mirrors, Grey 7, 159–167, 168, 196
  awareness, primordial energy of *11*
  life energy system *9*
  nervous system *8*
  personal narrative 161
  psychic energy system *10*, 161
  void/clear light *4*

The sacred and the soul, loss of 86
Sacred unconsciousness, Smith 153
Salaries, low 45
Sarter
  nursing therapeutics within consciousness
      paradigm 228–229
  visualization or imagery 229
Sarup, postmodern discourse 21
Schlitz, intentionality 119
Science and spirit 108
Scientific knowledge model, perpetuation by
    academic world 70
Sea metaphor, Chardin 5
Secular and sacred, balance between **79**
Self-knowledge 117
Sensory deprivation 215, 217
Separatist ontology 97
Shamanic cultures, view of illness 197
Shared consciousness 118
Shepherd
  sacred feminine ontology in transpersonal
      relationships 231–232
  Yin-Yang system, explanation 75–76
Shiatsu 216
Smell
  and healing, aromatherapy 249
  involuntary memories 213
Smith
  modern/postmodern juncture 8–9
  the sacred unconsciousness 153
Socialization
  and isolation of nursing xxii, 36
  and sexism, stereotypes 35
The soul 149–150
  soul work 150–151
Spear of Mars symbol 50
Spirit and science 108
Spiritual
  consciousness, Nightingale 264
  dimension, transpersonal caring-healing
      128
  perspective, importance 119
  practices, cultivating 148–149
  search for the 80
'Spiritual energy system', Grey, *Sacred Mirrors*
    10, 161
Steinbeck's boat 4
Steiner, anthroposophy 250
Stereotype to archetype 33–46
Stereotypes, nurses and women 33–34
  media 34–35
Steven, metaphor and metamorphosis 270
Subjectivity/intersubjectivity, sacred feminine
    archetype 232
Subtle biological energy, Benor 124
Sumer, ancient culture 60
Sweden, ontological shift, nursing education
    and practice 187

Symbol
  male and female 49, 50
  of nursing 34
  and ritual, reconsideration of 258–259

Tactile modality, intentional conscious use of
  214–218
  postmodern/transpersonal caring arts
    214–218
  premodern Nightingale 214–215
Tarnas
  covolution 54, 55
  crisis of culture as crisis of man 49, 50,
    51–52
  human experience 13
  The Passion of the Western Mind 69–70
Technical view, nursing 71
Telepathic messages, Bronte 139–140,
  141–142
Text to margin, moving 4–5, 17–22
Texture
  therapeutic use, sensory deprivation
    215, 217
  use in healing environment 253
Thailand, ontological shift, nursing education
  and practice 188
Theory-guided practice, benefits 186
Therapeutic
  massage 216
  presence 226
  touch 100, 124, 217
    additional modalities **223–224**
    modes and definitions 216
Thermal comfort, healing environment 252
Thomas
  the olfactory receptor cell 213–214
  view of music 208
Three Guineas, Woolf 66–67
Touch 229
  extrasensory perceptual abilities 144–145
  healing 217–218
  sensory deprivation 215, 217
  significance 67
  therapies *see* Therapeutic: touch
Toulmin
  modernity as worldview 247
  postmodern architecture 245
Trager **224**
Transformative
  capacity 144–146
  consciouness 128
  model of caring and healing 102
Transpersonal 290–291
  architecture 254
  body, exercises for experiencing 171–175
  caring
    see also Caring: moment

  connection 155
  discovery of human self 117
  model 154–157
  relationship 154–155
  caring-healing 105–130
    arts, use as technical interventions 228
    Era III/Paradigm III model 102–104
    modalities 206–227
    model xxii, 129–130
    paradigm xxv, xxvi
    premises 105–109
  consciousness, mind-body research
    123–128
  definition 115
  model
    of caring, requirement 180
    premises 179–180
  phase of awareness 103–104
  practice, professional ontological
    competencies 177–200
  presence 226
  relationships, sacred feminine archetype
    231–232
  self, cultivation of 227
Transpersonal/postmodern *see*
  Postmodern/transpersonal
Twenty-first century thinking 94

UK, ontological shift, nursing education and
  practice 183, 188
Unitary consciousness 180
Unitary-transformative paradigm *see*
  Paradigms: nursing: paradigm III
Universal unconscious and the sacred
  unconscious 151–153
University of Colorado Center for Human
  Caring 7, 189–192, 275–276
  international affiliate activities 191
  published information 189–190
Urban issues, rethinking 52–53
USA, ontologically based nursing practices
  and scholarship 183–185

Values 97
  see also Moral
  ontological shift in 104
  postmodern crisis 68
  re-evaluation of white, middle class
    17–18
  values-based approach 263
Venus's mirror 49–56
  journal entry 62–63
  a new looking glass 87–88
Views of nature, healing environment 253
Vipassana meditation 137–138
Virtual space and cyberspace 142–143

Visual modalities, intentional conscious use of 209–212
  postmodern/transpersonal caring arts 210–212
  premodern Nightingale 209–210
Visualization 211, 229

Walker, Margaret 3
War
  how do we prevent 62, 64
  medicine as 57, 58
  mythologies, Western literature 69
Watkins, negative emotions 124
Watson, deconstructing the modern 95
Western
  cultural cosmology 15
  intellect and spiritual being, covolution 54
  intellectual tradition, male perspective 50–51
  medicine, lack of feminine viewpoint 14–16
  mind, epochal shift 56
  scientific tradition, attack on 69
Whitehead, concrescence 114, 117
Wilber
  the body and consciousness 133–134
  meditation for the transpersonal self 167–168
Wolfe, modern architectural movement 245–247
Woman
  see also The feminine; The sacred feminine
  in ancient cultures 60–61
  and nurse as archtype 1, 80

Women
  and the professions, Woolf 66–67
  and society, Nightingale 66
Woolf, Three Guineas 66–67
Worldview
  evolving 2
  postmodern/transpersonal nursing requiring new 93
Writing as process of change xx

Yang
  definition 28, 291
  masculine principle 77
  themes, Epoch II, Kech's epochal evolution 81
Yin
  definition 291
  feminine principle 77
  themes, Epoch III, Kech's epochal evolution 82
Yin-Yang system 75–76

Zen
  of bedmaking 237–240
  definition 238
Zukav
  consciousness, energy and light, relationship 111–113, 121, 146, 147, 148, 256
  experience as non-physical light 143
  the extrasensory human 140–141
  intentionality 147
  reconsideration of physical/non physical 146
  the soul 149–150, 150–51